Varro E. Tyler, PhD, ScD

Herbs of Choice: The Therapeutic Use of Phytomedicinals

Pre-publication REVIEWS, COMMENTARIES, EVALUATIONS . . .

"**H**ERBS OF CHOICE CAT-APULTS HERBAL MEDICINE FROM FOLKLORE INTO MAIN-STREAM MEDICINE. Varro Tyler succinctly states not only what works and why an herb works, but how it works best. Amidst the myriad of herb books, Tyler has produced *the* practical volume of reliable information for health care practitioners. It is the only book in the herb advocacy literature that advocates a scientific approach to the subject.

Dr. Tyler is well-known for his support of a rational approach to the use of herb products as drugs in modern health care. In *Herbs of Choice*, he explores the important issue of "the herb regulatory dilemma," and proposes a solution based on adoption of a modified version of the existing German therapeutic monograph model.

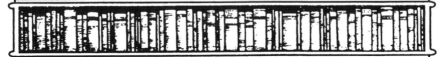

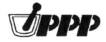

Pharmaceutical Products Press
An Imprint of The Haworth Press, Inc.

Herbs of Choice
The Therapeutic Use of Phytomedicinals

Herbs of Choice
The Therapeutic Use of Phytomedicinals

Varro E. Tyler, PhD, ScD

Lilly Distinguished Professor
of Pharmacognosy
Purdue University School of Pharmacy
and Pharmacal Sciences

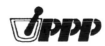

Pharmaceutical Products Press
An Imprint of the Haworth Press, Inc.
New York • London • Norwood (Australia)

Published by

Pharmaceutical Products Press, an imprint of The Haworth Press, Inc., 10 Alice Street, Binghamton, NY 13904-1580

The development, preparation, and publication of this work has been undertaken with great care. However, the publisher, employees, editors, and agents of The Haworth Press are not responsible for any errors contained herein or for consequences that may ensue from use of materials or information contained in this work. The opinions expressed by the author(s) are not necessarily those of The Haworth Press, Inc.

Library of Congress Cataloging-in-Publication Data

Tyler, Varro E.
    Herbs of choice : the therapeutic use of phytomedicinals / Varro E. Tyler.
        p.   cm.
    Includes bibliographical references and index.
    ISBN 1-56024-895-5 (acid-free paper).
    1. Herbs–Therapeutic use. I. Title.
RM666.H33T93   1994
615′.321–dc20   93-41977
                                                            CIP

For Michael and Anna–
you are my future!

ABOUT THE AUTHOR

Varro E. Tyler, PhD, ScD, a recognized authority on plant drugs (herbs) and their uses, is currently Lilly Distinguished Professor of Pharmacognosy in the School of Pharmacy and Pharmacal Sciences at Purdue University. He is the senior author of *Pharmacognosy, 9th Edition*, the standard U.S. textbook in the field, and *The Honest Herbal*, recently published by Pharmaceutical Products Press. Dr. Tyler is the author of over two hundred scientific and educational publications, including more than a dozen books, many of them dealing with pharmacognosy. He is a member of the editorial boards of several journals and a fellow of the Academy of Pharmaceutical Research and Science, the Academy of Pharmaceutical Scientists, and the American Association for the Advancement of Science, as well as an honorary member and past president of the American Society of Pharmacognosy. Dr. Tyler was Purdue University's executive vice-president for academic affairs for five years, and for twenty was Dean of its School of Pharmacy and Pharmacal Sciences.

CONTENTS

Preface

This book fills a long-existing gap in the English medical and pharmaceutical literature by providing, for the first time, essential information about the therapeutic use of the beneficial crude drugs of plant origin (herbs) and their common preparations (phytomedicinals). It does not discuss their folkloric or putative uses, nor does it dwell on unproven remedies with hoped-for attributes. Instead, it features current, factual information on a type of drug little-regarded presently by health care professionals in the United States but highly valued by their counterparts in other advanced nations, and in developing ones as well. A very few herbs of a nonbeneficial or toxic nature are mentioned briefly, primarily to contradict the abundant misinformation presently circulating concerning them.

In presenting the facts to the interested reader, I have fulfilled a decades-old dream of clearing, for professional and lay readers alike, a broad and level pathway through the minefield of hyperbole and hoax so often associated with herbal medicine in this country. Written at a professional level, the book will nevertheless benefit consumers by enabling physicians and other health professionals to prescribe or to recommend for them reasonably priced, effective medicines for many common ailments. Alternatively, it will permit the informed nonprofessional to self-select low-cost, useful remedies for certain minor afflictions. Such objectives are exceedingly important in this era of escalating health care costs.

It is never advisable to state that one's coverage of a subject is complete. Authors are human beings, and human beings sometimes err. But it is possible to say that this volume represents the first scientifically and clinically documented account in the English language of most of the truly useful herbs and phytomedicinals. Absence of a particular product may be taken as highly indicative that, at present, its therapeutic utility is unproven. Provision of information on only the therapeutically useful herbs–unless an exception is specifically noted–distinguishes this volume from almost all other herbal writings in which preliminary indications and wishful thinking combine to render them of little value.

Many persons have assisted greatly in the preparation of *Herbs of Choice*. Dr. Götz Harnischfeger kindly supplied me with copies of pertinent reports of the *Bundesgesundheitsamt* Commission E as published in the *Bundesanzeiger*. Mark Blumenthal continually provided references and copies of recently published herbal papers by means of his invaluable HerbClip service. Professor emerita Theodora Andrews exhaustively searched the vast health-related literature for useful information. My assistant, Linda Michael, computerized and recomputerized more versions of the developing manuscript than anyone will ever know. Ginny Tyler, long my wife but always much more, provided her customary excellent editorial assistance, in addition to preparing the detailed index. Thank you, one and all!

Chapter 1

Basic Principles

DEFINITIONS

Herbs are defined in several ways depending on the context in which the word is used. In botanical nomenclature, the word refers to non-woody seed-producing plants that die down at the end of the growing season. In the culinary arts, it refers to vegetable products used to add flavor or aroma to food. But in the field of medicine, the term has a different, yet specific, meaning. Here it is most accurately defined as **crude drugs of vegetable origin utilized for the treatment of disease states, often of a chronic nature, or to attain or maintain a condition of improved health**. Pharmaceutical preparations made by extracting herbs with various solvents to yield tinctures, fluidextracts, extracts, or the like, are known as phytomedicinals (plant medicines).

In the United States, the choice of an herb or phytomedicine for therapeutic or preventive purposes is usually carried out by the patient. To state it differently, the herb is self-selected. That is because physicians here are not ordinarily educated in the use of such medicinals. However, in many other countries, herbs and phytomedicinals are prescribed by doctors with considerable frequency.

It cannot be emphasized strongly enough that herbs in their medicinal sense are drugs. For reasons that will become apparent when the legal concerns regarding herbs are discussed in the next chapter, certain special interest groups continually emphasize their point of view that medicinal herbs are foods or nutritional supplements. That is not the case. If they are used in the treatment (cure or mitigation) of disease or improvement of health (diagnosis or prevention of disease), they conform to the definition of the word *drug*.

1

There are, however, a limited number of botanical products that may qualify either as foods or drugs or both, depending on the specific intent of the user. Employed as a flavoring agent in cooking, garlic is clearly a food. When it is used to control hypertension or high cholesterol levels, it is a drug. Possibly some may use it for both purposes at the same time. The millions of elderly Americans who drink prune juice daily probably consider it both a pleasant breakfast beverage (food) and a means of maintaining "regularity" (drug). Plantago (psyllium) seed also falls in this ambivalent category. Widely used on a daily basis as an over-the-counter (OTC) bulk laxative that can be purchased without a physician's prescription, the seed would be classified by most users as a drug. The same nutritious seed incorporated into a breakfast cereal is certainly nothing more than a healthful food.

The only way to settle this dilemma is to admit that a relatively few plant products defy precise definition as either foods or drugs. Fortunately, in the vast panoply of herbs, relatively few present this classificational problem. Those that do are mostly specialized storage organs of the plants, such as fruits, seeds, or fleshy underground parts rich in carbohydrates. The problem is much less frequently encountered with the flowering tops, leaves and stems, barks, rhizomes, and/or roots that constitute most herbs. The basic definition still applies. Herbs used for medicinal purposes are drugs.

DIFFERENCES BETWEEN HERBS AND OTHER DRUGS

Herbs are different in several respects from the type of purified therapeutic agents we have become accustomed to call *drugs* in the last half of the twentieth century. In the first place, they are more dilute than the concentrated chemicals that are familiar to us in the form of aspirin tablets or tetracycline capsules. A simple example will illustrate the difference. One can take caffeine for its stimulatory effects on the central nervous system. The usual dose is 200 mg. contained in one or two small tablets, depending on their strength. Or, it is possible to get the same effect by drinking a caffeine-containing beverage, such as coffee or tea. Because coffee normally contains 1 to 2 percent of the active constituent, it is necessary to extract up to 20 g. (2/3 ounce) of the product to yield that same amount. Tea contains more caffeine–up to 4 percent–but the method of preparation extracts less of it. Probably about 10 g. (1/3 ounce) of tea would be necessary to yield the same amount of caffeine found in 1 or 2 tablets. This assumes the beverage would be boiled during its preparation, rather than steeped as is the usual custom.[1]

Dilution is not the only difference that must be considered in utilizing medicinal herbs. In addition to physiologically inert substances such as cellulose and starch, herbs often contain additional active principles that may be closely related both chemically and therapeutically to the constituent primarily responsible for its effects. Digitalis is a much-cited example of just such an herb. Various species of this leafy herb contain some 30 different closely related glycosides, all of which possess cardiotonic properties but which, due to small structural differences, have different speeds of onset of action and different durations of their effects. For example, one of the glycosides, digitoxin, when administered orally has an onset of action of 1 to 4 hours with peak activity demonstrated at 8 to 14 hours. Another, digoxin, has an onset of action ranging from 1/2 to 2 hours and reaches a peak activity level in 2 to 6 hours.[2]

Certain digitalis plants contain both of these active principles along with many others. Proponents of the use of the whole leaf argue that it is a very effective and useful drug because its multiplicity of constituents provides a uniform activity of short onset and long duration. While this is true to some degree, it is also true that the activity of the leaf is difficult to standardize, which explains why it is seldom used in the United States. The presently employed procedure that involves cardiac arrest in pigeons is just one of a long series of biological assays utilizing such animals as frogs, cats, goldfish, chicks and even daphnia (water fleas) in an attempt to obtain an accurate measure of potency. The ability to measure physiological potency in terms of the weight of a pure chemical entity is one of the principal reasons why administration of a purified constituent was considered advantageous in the first place. This concept is not new. It dates back to Paracelsus in the early sixteenth century.[3]

In addition to containing constituents with a desired activity, herbs often contain other principles that detract from their specific therapeutic utility. For example, cinchona bark contains some 25 related alkaloids, but the only one recognized as useful in the treatment of malaria is quinine. Thus, if powdered cinchona bark is administered as a treatment for malaria, the patient will also receive appreciable amounts of the alkaloid quinidine, a cardiac depressant, and cinchotannic acid, which because of its astringent properties would induce constipation.[4] Such side effects must be taken into account in the use of medicinal herbs.

HERBAL QUALITY

The matter of proper identification and appropriate quality, that is, lack of adulteration, sophistication, or substitution, is an extremely important one in the field of herbal medicine. Many of today's widely used herbs were once the subject of official monographs in *The United States Pharmacopeia* (*USP*) and *The National Formulary* (*NF*). These monographs established legal standards of identity and, subject to the limitations of the methods of the period, of quality of the vegetable drugs.

No such standards exist today. Many of the herbs sold in the U.S. are collected in the wild in developing nations by persons who are not necessarily knowledgeable about the subtleties of plant taxonomy. The herbs are then sold to organizations that usually market them under their common names instead of their recognized Latin binomials; this can cause confusion because of the lack of uniformity of the common names. Likewise, the marketer may not employ the necessary skilled personnel nor have the requisite analytical equipment to be able to establish identity and quality of the wide variety of botanicals sold. Herbs are sold in various ways ranging from essentially whole plants or plant parts to cut pieces to finely ground powders. It is ordinarily impossible for the lay person to determine the quality or even the identity of the plant material by visual inspection. Because government standards of quality are nonexistent in the United States, the buyer is totally dependent upon the reputation of the seller. As a general rule, the larger firms have more to lose if they sell herbs of inferior quality, but some smaller organizations have outstanding reputations for marketing quality materials.

Returning to the matter of standardization of herbs or herbal extracts, it must be noted that the concentration of active constituents in different lots of supposedly identical plant material is highly variable. First of all, genetic variations exist. Just as one variety of apple tree will produce larger or tastier apples than another, so too will one variety of peppermint produce a larger quantity or a more flavorful peppermint oil than another, even though the conditions of growth remain identical. These genetic variations in medicinal herbs, many of which are obtained from wild-growing plants, are not well understood.

Also of great importance to the quality of an herb are the environmental conditions under which it is grown. Fertility of the soil, length of growing season, temperature, amount of moisture, and time of harvest are some of the significant factors. Processing also plays a role. Some constituents are heat labile, and the plant material containing them needs to be dried at low temperatures. Other active principles are destroyed by enzymatic processes that continue for long periods of time if the herb is dried too slowly.

Since few of these factors are precisely controlled even for cultivated plants, let alone those harvested from the wild, the most effective way to assure herbal quality is to assay, that is, to establish by some means the amount of active constituent(s) in the plant material. If the chemical identity of the constituent is known, it usually can be isolated and quantified by appropriate physical or chemical methods. If it is unknown or if it is a complex mixture of constituents, a biological assay such as that employed for digitalis must be utilized. Once the potency of the herb is known, it can be mixed with appropriate quantities of material of greater or lesser potency to produce a product with defined activity. At the present time, standardization of medicinal herbs is still uncommon.

In terms of quality, the more expensive the plant material, the more likely it is to be inferior. Finely powdered herbs, or dosage forms such as tablets or capsules made from them, are particularly susceptible to fraud by adulteration or substitution. One study of 54 ginseng products showed that 60 percent of those analyzed were worthless and 25 percent of them contained no ginseng at all.[5] A recent Canadian study showed that no North American feverfew product analyzed contained the recommended minimal content of

0.2 percent parthenolide believed to be required for effectiveness.[6] For many years, the root of prairie dock, *Parthenium integrifolium* L., was wrongly marketed as echinacea (*Echinacea* spp.),[7] and may still be in some isolated instances. Volatile-oil-containing botanicals often have their aromas enhanced by the addition of quantities of essential oils from other sources. This is said to be a common practice in the beverage herbal tea industry.

Although standardized extracts of ginkgo, ginseng, milk thistle, St. John's wort, and a few other plants are available, the quality of most herbs in the American market today is extremely variable. This presents a problem because it makes the establishment of a specific dose difficult, if not impossible. It would be more of a problem if it were not for the fact that the therapeutic potency and potential toxicity of the active principles in many herbs are very modest, and this, when coupled with the great dilution in which they occur in the plant material, usually renders precise dosage unnecessary.

It is also this lack of high therapeutic potency that makes herbs more useful for the long-term treatment of mild or chronic complaints than for the rapid healing of acute illnesses. This is well illustrated in the current usage of feverfew as a preventive in cases of migraine or vascular headache. While the herb has no utility in the treatment of acute attacks, accumulated evidence indicates its effectiveness in preventing such attacks if taken on a regular basis.[8]

PARAHERBALISM

Belief in the superiority of things natural and organic, which gained considerable impetus in the United States in recent decades, may be viewed as an outgrowth of the counterculture movement of the 1960s. It has been perpetuated largely by people who are well intentioned but who are ignorant of many of the basic principles of science. In 1828, Friedrich Wöhler's synthesis of urea from inorganic starting materials laid to rest, once and for all, the doctrine of vitalism. Yet, in this last decade of the twentieth century, we still find persons insisting that vitamin C from natural sources is in some way different from and superior to vitamin C prepared synthetically from glucose.

"Organic" has taken on a special meaning with respect to plant products and now refers to materials, including herbs, grown without the use of synthetic pesticides or synthetic fertilizers. While no one wants to ingest plant material appreciably contaminated with foreign toxicants, the Environmental Protection Agency has established residue "tolerance" standards to prevent this. Further, it is now well-known that a large number of toxicants, especially carcinogens, are present naturally in commonly consumed foods ranging from apples to tomatoes.[9] In all likelihood, the accumulation of such natural poisons serves to protect the plant from predators, thereby assisting its evolutionary survival. As for the merits of natural versus synthetic fertilizers, plants are totally unable to differentiate the origin of required nutritional elements, so only the presence or the lack thereof, not the nature of the source, is of significance.

In spite of the absence of scientific proof regarding the superiority of "natural" medicines, there are still those today who, in support of the belief that herbs have mystical, even magical properties, have turned their type of herbalism into a pseudoscience. I have previously referred to such persons as paraherbalists and their concept of herbalism as paraherbalism.[10] The ten tenets or precepts that distinguish paraherbalism from rational herbalism (only one of which deals with the natural versus synthetic issue) are worthy of presenting here in summarized form. Awareness of them will assist interested persons in distinguishing fact from fiction in a field where the former is scarce and the latter is abundant. Proceed with caution any time one of the following italicized statements appears in an herbal reference work or journal article.

1. *A conspiracy by the medical establishment discourages the use of herbs.* There is no conspiracy. Very few health care practitioners have any knowledge of the field because the subject is not included in most academic curricula. The pharmaceutical industry generally views phytomedicinals as unprofitable products.
2. *Herbs cannot harm, only cure.* Some of the most toxic substances known–amatoxins, convallatoxin, aconitine, strychnine, abrin, ricin–are derived from plants.

3. *Whole herbs are more effective than their isolated active constituents.* For every example cited in support of this thesis, there is at least one example denying it. Besides, many herbs contain toxins in addition to useful principles. Comfrey is an example.

4. *"Natural" and "organic" herbs are superior to synthetic drugs.* As previously noted, Wöhler disproved the "natural" part of this in 1828. Established limits on pesticide residues render treated plants no more harmful than "organic" plants.

5. *The Doctrine of Signatures is meaningful.* This ancient belief postulates that the form of a plant part determines its therapeutic virtue. If it were true, kidney beans should cure all types of renal disease and walnuts should cure various types of cerebral malfunction.

6. *Reducing the dose of a medicine increases its therapeutic activity.* There is no proof that this is generally true, as espoused by practitioners of homeopathy. Positive results obtained by homeopathic treatment are demonstrations of the placebo effect.

7. *Astrological influences are significant.* No scientific evidence supports this assertion.

8. *Physiological tests in animals are not applicable to human beings.* Differences do exist, but there is a high probability of significance and applicability when diverse animal species, especially those from different orders, show similar effects.

9. *Anecdotal evidence is highly significant.* It is extremely difficult to assess the reliability of such evidence. Consequently, it must be viewed simply as one of many factors (animal tests, clinical trials, etc.) that may tend to indicate the therapeutic utility of an herb.

10. *Herbs were created by God specifically to cure disease.* This thesis is not testable and should not be used as a substitute for scientific evidence.

Unfortunately, the practitioners of paraherbalism who espouse one or more of these tenets have done much to discredit the legitimate use of herbs for therapeutic purposes. For whatever reason, be it misguided belief, personal gain, or simply ignorance, they have flooded the market with literature containing so much outdated and downright inaccurate information about the use of herbs that interested individuals, lay or professional, who approach the field for the first time become totally confused. Because it serves their purposes, paraherbalists often accept at face value the disproven positive statements of a Renaissance herbalist such as Nicholas Culpeper[11] or a folk writer such as Maria Treben,[12] but discount the findings of modern science that demonstrate the toxicity of an herbal product.[13]

RATIONAL HERBALISM

All of this has done much to discredit herbal medicine, and those seeking to establish its validity start with a severe handicap. Nevertheless, a knowledge of historical drug development will indicate immediately that plants have long served as useful and rational sources of therapeutic agents. Not only do plant drugs such as digitalis, the opium poppy, ergot, cinchona bark, plantago seed, cascara sagrada, rauwolfia, belladonna, coca leaves, and others continue to serve as useful sources of pharmaceuticals, their constituents also serve as models for many of the synthetic drugs used in modern medicine. It is not unreasonable to expect that of the 13,000 plant species that are known to have been used as drugs throughout the world, some of them literally for centuries, there are still many with useful therapeutic properties that have been little studied.[14] Thus, while we may as yet be unable to isolate, purify, and market a botanical's chemical constituent for use as a drug, the herb that contains it may still be used in its natural or phytomedicinal form, and desirable therapeutic effects may be achieved.

It is, therefore, important to realize that while herbs are literally diluted drugs, the nature of the active principle(s) in them is often a matter of empirical observation and tradition rather than the result of extensive clinical testing. The reasons for this lack of clinical testing are basically economic, for the cost of such evaluation is extremely high.

However, perhaps even more important than whether an herbal remedy works, i.e., has the desired therapeutic utility, is the matter of whether it is safe. It might be surmised that herbs consumed by humans for generations, centuries, and even millennia must be rea-

sonably safe. This has generally proven true, at least insofar as
acute toxicity is concerned. But it is not necessarily true for some of
the newly introduced, more exotic products that are continually
being placed on the market by herbal enthusiasts. Nor is it the case
for some of the older herbs that have recently been shown to produce deleterious effects of a chronic, more subtle nature following
long usage. Certain comfrey species with their content of toxic
pyrrolizidine alkaloids are an excellent example of this latter kind
of herb.[15]

Some have questioned the validity of herbal medicine because
they doubt the wisdom of self-treatment for diseases of any kind,
and as previously noted, most herbal treatments in this country are
self-selected. That this point of view is largely invalid is obvious to
anyone who has followed the recent trend in over-the-counter
(OTC) drugs. A number of significant drugs, including hydrocortisone, ibuprofen, clotrimazole, and various antihistamines have been
converted recently from prescription to OTC status, and this trend is
continuing.

What is important with respect to self-medication is knowing
which conditions to treat and which ones deserve professional medical care. The occasional pain of a headache or a strained muscle, a
mild digestive upset or simple diarrhea, infrequent insomnia, the
common cold–all are conditions that are amenable to, and usually
receive, self-treatment. On the other hand, a sufferer from rheumatoid arthritis, cardiac arrythmia, or cancer requires professional
medical care. Self-treatment in such conditions would be utter folly.

Many books dealing with "unconventional" or "alternative"
medicine contain, along with discourses on such subjects as acupuncture and homeopathy, a chapter or two on herbal medicine.
This shows a complete lack of understanding on the part of the
authors of such reference works. **Rational herbal medicine is conventional medicine**. It is merely the application of diluted drugs to
the prevention and cure of disease. The fact that the constituents
and, sometimes, even the mode of action of these drugs are often
incompletely understood and that instruction in their appropriate
application is not a significant part of standard medical curricula
does not in any way detract from their role in conventional medicine. If it did, we would be forced to discontinue the use of a

number of popular products such as plantago seed and senna laxatives, together with about 25 percent of our current materia medica that is derived from such sources. We would also have to conclude that some 52 percent of all German adults are unconventional because this is the percentage who turn first to a natural remedy (herbs or phytomedicines) to treat their illnesses.[16] Chinese medicine has become a hybrid of Western and traditional practices, but personal observation indicates that if the use of herbal medicine were considered unconventional, almost the entire population of China would fall into this category. Although herbal therapy may not be mainstream American medicine, it certainly is conventional.

Confusion between herbal medicine and homeopathy may exist in the minds of many persons because herbs are frequently used by homeopathic practitioners. It is useful to note that the philosophical contexts of the two are completely different, and although they may employ the same basic remedies, the way in which they are used is also completely different. Homeopathy is based on the untenable hypothesis that decreasing the dose of a drug increases the physiological response to it. As a matter of fact, its proponents argue that the dose may be decreased to the point where the drug is no longer present, but the diluent (milk sugar, water and/or alcohol, etc.) in which the drug was once present will remain extremely potent. There is no reliable scientific or clinical evidence that confirms the validity of homeopathy.[17] It must never be confused with herbal medicine, for the two are completely unrelated.

HERBAL DOSAGE FORMS

Herbs are consumed in various ways, most commonly in the form of a tea or tisane prepared from the dried plant material. Both of these terms refer to what is technically known as an infusion, prepared by pouring boiling water over the herb and allowing it to steep for a period of time. In such cases, the herb and the water are not boiled together. Time of steeping is important, for many of the desired components are not very water soluble. For example, in the case of chamomile where much of the desired activity is present in the volatile oil, even a prolonged steeping of 10 minutes extracts only about 10 to 15 percent of the desired components.[18]

Occasionally an herbal preparation is made by boiling the plant material in water for a period of time, then straining and drinking the resulting extract. Technically, the process is called decocting, and the resulting liquid is known as a decoction. Boiled coffee is prepared in this way as opposed to beverage tea, which is an infusion.

The quantity of herb to be extracted is usually rather imprecise, being stated in terms of level or heaping teaspoonfuls. A standard teaspoonful of water weighs about 5 grams (approximately 1/6 ounce), and a heaping teaspoonful of most herbal materials weighs approximately half that (2.5 g.). Very light herbs, such as the flower heads that comprise chamomile, may weigh only 1.0 g. per heaping teaspoonful. The same quantity of a leaf drug might weigh 1.5 g., and of a root or bark about 4.5 g. Even these weights are variable according to the degree of comminution (chopping or grinding) of the plant material. Finely powdered herbs are obviously going to have less space among the particles, and an equal volume will weigh more. A heaping teaspoonful of finely powdered ginger weighs about 5 g. Standard instructions for the preparation of a tea call for one heaping teaspoonful per cup of water (240 ml. or 8 fluidounces). It must be noted the stated sizes of teaspoons are those established by long-standing convention. Experience indicates that modern teaspoons have a capacity some 25 percent greater than these standards.[19] For most herbal preparations this difference is probably of minor significance.

The volume of a standard cup as described in this work (240 ml.) is that of the common household measure, not the pharmaceutical teacup, which contains only half that quantity, 120 ml. (4 fluidounces). The latter measurement is little known or used, even by modern-day professionals, to say nothing of lay consumers. In many European herbal writings, the figure 150 ml. is employed as a convenient amount of water to use for the preparation of various herb teas. That figure is also cited in some of the monographs that follow, which were derived from the German literature. As was the case with the teaspoonful measurements just cited, these variations in the size of cupfuls are relatively unimportant. What is important is to use a sufficient volume of water to extract thoroughly the active constituents from the quantity of plant material employed.

As previously noted, herbs are often marketed as phytomedicinals in various dosage forms. Some of the more common ones include powders in hard gelatin capsules or, together with suitable fillers and binders, as compressed tablets. When the active principles are not soluble in water or when a more concentrated product is required to allow adequate dosage, various extracts of herbs are prepared. These are usually hydroalcoholic solutions or tinctures of such concentration that 10 ml. will contain the active constituents in either 1 or 2 g. of herb. Even more concentrated preparations are known as fluidextracts, 1 ml. of which represents 1 g. of plant material. Tinctures or fluidextracts are consumed as such or by diluting a specific quantity–usually a certain number of drops–in water so that they may be easily swallowed. The most concentrated form of an herb is a solid extract prepared by evaporating all of the solvent used to remove the active constituents from the herb. Extracts are often available in powdered form; 1 g. usually represents 2-8 g. of the starting material. They are normally encapsulated for ease in administration.

If consumers do decide to purchase the herbs themselves, rather than a processed dosage form, they should remember certain guidelines that will help assure the acquisition of a quality product. Lacking expert knowledge, however, there is no sure way to avoid all of the pitfalls. Buying clean, dried herbs that are as fresh as possible from a reputable source, preferably in a form allowing positive identification, and assuring freedom from insect infestation by careful inspection, is probably the best general advice. Many herbs are valued for their aromatic principles. These are stable in whole plant parts for a longer period of time than in finely powdered material. Such plant parts can easily be reduced to the desired fineness in a small electric coffee grinder just before making a tea. Maintain all herbs in tightly closed, preferably glass containers, away from sunlight, and in a cool, dry place.

These, then, are the basic principles of herbal medicine as they apply to its current practice in the United States. The field is a curious mixture of ancient tradition applied to modern conditions without, in many cases, the benefit of modern science and technology. To be totally effective, the traditional practices must eventually be coupled with up-to-date scientific methodology. The reason that has not yet been done, except in certain isolated circum-stances, will become clear in the next chapter, which examines the present laws and regulations pertaining to herbs in this country.

The cooperation between empiricism and science, so urgently needed to bring herbs and phytomedicines into the mainstream of modern medicine, is a subject that has been explored in some depth by B. Lehmann, a German physician. Her conclusion, given here in translation, is especially pertinent and serves as a fitting summary to this chapter on "Basic Principles":[20]

> Phytomedicines, exactly like other medicines, must stand up to the challenge of modern scientific evaluation. They need no special consideration when it comes to the planning and con-duct of clinical trials intended to prove their safety and effi-cacy. The distinctive feature of phytotherapy is its origin, namely, the many years of empirical use of plant drugs. Expe-rience gained during this period should be taken into account, along with clinical testing, in evaluating the effectiveness of phytomedicines.

REFERENCE NOTES

1. Tyler, V.E.: *The Honest Herbal*, 3rd ed., Pharmaceutical Products Press, Binghamton, New York, 1993, pp. 69-72.

2. Tyler, V.E., Brady, L.R., and Robbers, J.E.: *Pharmacognosy*, 9th ed., Lea & Febiger, Philadelphia, 1988, pp. 164-171.

3. Sonnedecker, G.: *Kremers and Urdang's History of Pharmacy*, 4th ed., J.B. Lippincott Company, Philadelphia, 1976, pp. 40-42.

4. Tyler, V.E., Brady, L.R., and Robbers, J.E.: *Pharmacognosy*, 9th ed., Lea & Febiger, Philadelphia, 1988, pp. 204, 208.

5. Ziglar, W.: *Whole Foods* **2**(4): 48-53 (1979).

6. Awang, D.V.C., Dawson, B.A., Kindack, D.G., Crompton, C.W., and Hep-tinstall, S.: *Journal of Natural Products* **54**:1516-1521 (1991).

7. Foster, S.: *Echinacea: Nature's Immune Enhancer*, Healing Arts Press, Rochester, Vermont, 1991, pp. 84-92.

8. Hobbs, C.: *HerbalGram* No. 20:30-33 (1989).

9. Abelson, P.: *Science* **249**:1357 (1990).

10. Tyler, V.E.: *Nutrition Forum* **6**:41-44 (1989).

11. Culpeper, N.: *Culpeper's Complete Herbal and English Physician En-larged*, Richard Evans, London, 1814, 398 pp.

12. Treben, M.: *Health Through God's Pharmacy*, Wilhelm Ennsthaler, Steyr, Austria, 1980, 88 pp.

13. Heinerman, J.: *The Science of Herbal Medicine*, Bi-World Publishers, Orem, Utah, 1979, xvi-xxi.

14. Dragendorff, G.: *Die Heilpflanzen der verschiedenen Völker und Zeiten*, Ferdinand Enke, Stuttgart, 1898, 885 pp.

15. Awang, D.V.C.: *Canadian Pharmaceutical Journal* **120**:100-104 (1987).

16. Tyler, V.E.: *Nutrition Forum* **1**:11 (1984).

17. Barrett, S.: *Nutrition Forum* **4**:1-6 (1987).

18. Tyler, V.E., Brady, L.R., and Robbers, J.E.: *Pharmacognosy*, 9th ed., Lea & Febiger, Philadelphia, 1988, pp. 466-467.

19. Lowenthal, W. and Goldstein, S.W.: "Metrology and Calculation," in *Remington's Pharmaceutical Sciences*, 16th ed., A. Osol, ed., Mack Publishing Company, Easton, Penn., 1980, pp. 73-74.

20. Lehmann, B.: *Zeitschrift für Phytotherapie* **13**:14-18 (1992).

Chapter 2

The Herbal Regulatory Dilemma

A REGULATORY TOWER OF BABEL

Persons involved today in the legal regulation of drugs, especially those in the herbal category, must look back to the latter years of the nineteenth century with a real sense of nostalgia. All things were clearer then–black was black and white was white. Ginseng, for example, was definitely a drug. Carefully monographed and described in *The United States Pharmacopeia* until 1882, it was perfectly permissible to label ginseng as a useful stimulant and stomachic. The drug was also widely employed in Chinese medicine as an aphrodisiac. Knowledgeable pharmacists who sold ginseng to the public could inform patrons in detail about the product, having studied it in detail as part of formal training.

As we approach the end of the twentieth century, black and white are seldom seen; gray abounds. Exactly what ginseng is depends to a large extent on where and of whom you inquire about it. Ask a Food and Drug Administration official in the United States, and you will be told that, legally, ginseng is a food for beverage use only, with no proven therapeutic values, especially in the area of increasing sexual potency. Inquire about it from a practitioner of traditional medicine in China, and you will be told that ginseng is a medicine with "positive action as a nerve and cardiac stimulant, increasing metabolism, retarding impotence, regulating blood pressure and blood sugar."[1] It is indicated in a variety of conditions ranging from asthma to rheumatism. In Germany, Switzerland, and most other countries of Western Europe, ginseng is widely promoted and sold as an over-the-counter drug, the beneficial effects of which are said to be primarily adaptogenic in nature. Australian

17

authorities classify ginseng as a therapeutic substance of a type presenting low or moderate risk to the consumer. Traditional claims of efficacy are allowed, provided certain general advertising requirements are met. In Canada, ginseng, like many other herbal products, is sold as a food with the understanding that it will generally be used for medicinal purposes. In France, recently implemented regulations permit the herb to be sold without the need for any toxicological studies. As long as ginseng is labeled as being traditionally used for transitory weakness, no clinical evaluation is deemed necessary either.

A casual observer might well wonder how this herbal Tower of Babel ever came to exist. Certainly no one would purposely plan it in such a way, and, of course, no one did. It seems to have come about because well-meaning regulators applied twentieth century standards to nineteenth century drugs–drugs which had originally been introduced into use as a result of long folkloric usage and accumulation of anecdotal evidence. When the standards of randomized, double-blind, cross-over clinical trials were applied to these ancient remedies, suddenly they did not fit in the system. In order to understand the system, it is necessary to examine its origins.

DRUG REGULATION 1906-1962

Early in this century, fraud was rampant among the producers of both foods and drugs in the United States. Harvey W. Wiley, then chief of the Bureau of Chemistry of the U.S. Department of Agriculture, undertook a vigorous campaign against the unscrupulous practices of both industries. His work resulted in passage of the Food and Drugs Act of 1906. This act, commonly but incorrectly referred to as the "Pure" Food and "Drug" Act, was at the time a true innovation. It, and the 1912 Sherley amendment to it, put an end to many fraudulent practices, such as the misbranding and adulteration of drugs, but failed to address effectively the problems of drug safety and efficacy.[2,3] Little attention was paid to such matters for more than 30 years, when a tragedy brought drug safety concerns to the fore.

The S.E. Massengill Company of Bristol, Tennessee, began to

market in 1937 an Elixir Sulfanilamide consisting of 8.8 percent of the drug in 72 percent diethylene glycol. This product, intended primarily for Southerners who liked to drink their medicines, was marketed without adequate toxicity testing in animals; in fact, it was tested only for flavor prior to marketing. Before the poisonous character of the solvent was recognized and the product could be recalled, it caused some 105 deaths resulting from acute kidney failure.[4] The public outcry resulting from this unfortunate episode precipitated the passage of the 1938 Federal Food, Drug, and Cosmetic Act. Among its requirements was one necessitating that drugs entering interstate commerce be proven safe. If a drug already on the market was subject to the 1906 Act, it was grandfathered, and additional proof of safety was not required.

Although a number of amendments were made to the 1938 Act, including a rather significant one (Durham-Humphrey) in 1951 which dealt largely with classification and procedures, it took another tragedy to bring about substantial change. Thalidomide, a sedative drug developed by Chemie Grünenthal G.m.b.H. in Stolberg, Germany, in 1953 and widely marketed in Europe, was identified in 1962 as a potent teratogen. About 30-40 percent of the mothers who took the drug during a critical phase of their pregnancies gave birth to physically deformed babies. The drug was never marketed in the United States, but its observed side effects caused great concern here.[5]

This period of alarm coincided with an extensive Congressional investigation of the American drug industry led by Senator Estes Kefauver of Tennessee. All of these events resulted in the passage of the Drug Amendments of 1962, often referred to as the Kefauver-Harris Amendments. These required, among other things, that all drugs marketed in the United States after 1962 be proven *both safe and effective*. Again, drugs marketed prior to 1938 were grandfathered, but every product introduced between 1938 and 1962 was subject to these requirements. This group consisted of approximately 300 different chemical entities in about 4,000 different drug formulations that were actively being sold, and another 3,000 formulations that had been approved by the standard New Drug Application (NDA) process but were not actively marketed.

IMPLEMENTING SAFETY AND EFFICACY REGULATIONS

In view of the enormity of the task of evaluating the safety and efficacy of all these products, the federal Food and Drug Administration (FDA) turned for help to the Division of Medical Sciences of the National Academy of Sciences–National Research Council. They proceeded to organize a Drug Efficacy Study that began work in 1962. After a long series of preliminary investigations which lasted until 1969, 17 panels, each of which concerned itself with a different therapeutic class of drugs, were formed in 1972 to examine over-the-counter (OTC) drugs. This is the category in which most herbs and herb products would normally be classified.

The panels did not utilize all sources of information because some, such as patient testimonials, anecdotal experiences of physicians, and market success of the product, were considered unreliable. Instead, they relied primarily on in-vitro tests (studies not conducted in patients or whole animals) and on various kinds of clinical or patient trials. The panels themselves did not conduct these studies but only evaluated information supplied to them by organizations interested in marketing the drugs.

It was obviously impossible to examine the approximately one-third million drug products in the OTC category, so evaluations were limited to the active ingredients in them. Because of the paucity of information resulting from in-vitro tests or clinical trials with herbs, the panels were asked to evaluate a relatively small number of such drugs, and then only for specific indications. Besides, most of them had apparently been grandfathered under both the 1938 and 1962 Acts and were considered immune from the *effective* requirements implemented at the later date.

FDA'S HERBAL REGULATORY INITIATIVE

Nevertheless, the FDA undertook the regulation of herbs by what can only be termed an extremely innovative application of administrative law. The agency simply declared that any of the grandfathered drugs would be considered misbranded and subject to confiscation if any claims of efficacy were made for them which were not in accordance with the findings of one of the 17 OTC drug evaluation panels. Thus, it became possible to sell the product only if no claims or statements regarding its value in the prevention or treatment of disease were made on the label. The word *label* is very broadly defined to include not only the words on the package itself but also those on any accompanying literature, such as a package insert. In this way, herbs were effectively prevented from being marketed as the drugs many of them are.

Results of the FDA study of OTC drugs were finally released to the public in the spring of 1990.[6] Although some of the herbs, including cascara bark and senna leaf, were found to be effective (in these cases, as laxatives) and placed in category I, some 258 non-prescription drug ingredients, many of them herbs, were not so judged. Of these, 142 were categorized as unsafe or ineffective (category II), and there was insufficient evidence to evaluate the effectiveness of the other 116. These were placed in Category III. Again, the panels made these judgments only on the basis of evidence submitted to them by the industry, and as a result, there are some surprises in their listings. Peppermint oil was included in Category III, being found ineffective as a digestive aid due to lack of evidence, and the same reasoning was applied to prune concentrate and powder, which were classified as ineffective laxatives.

From the scientific viewpoint, it is extremely difficult to defend the compartmentalized thinking that led to these particular decisions. Denying, for whatever reason, the effectiveness of products that everyone knows are effective, and which could be verified by simple experimentation–such as drinking a glass or two of prune juice–is perverse. Unwarranted and obviously incorrect categorizations of this sort place in jeopardy the credibility of the entire OTC review procedure.

REACTION TO FDA'S HERBAL REGULATIONS

Reaction of the herb industry to the FDA's stricture on therapeutic labeling of products judged to be ineffective by the panels took a variety of forms. Some herbs ceased to be marketed. Others continued to be sold as before, in the hope that an underfunded and overworked FDA might overlook, at least for a period of time, some of the infractions. But the most frequent course of action was simply to remove the offending information from the label and to market the product as a food, nutritional supplement, or in some cases, as a food additive. Unfortunately, this left little on the label except the name of the herb. For some time, the FDA has maintained a list of substances "Generally Recognized as Safe," better known in the trade as the GRAS list.[7] About 250 herbs appear on this list primarily based on their use as food additives, that is, as flavors or spices in the culinary arts and the beverage industry. Some of them, such as ginger and glycyrrhiza, are also employed for their medicinal action. Obviously, if a plant material is simply labeled "ginger," it is impossible to know whether it will be used as a food additive (flavor) or as a medicine to prevent motion sickness. Perhaps in some cases, ginger from the same package would be used both ways.

The FDA formerly maintained two other lists in addition to the GRAS list. These were "Herbs of Undefined Safety" and a list of 27 "Unsafe Herbs." Both were flawed by inappropriate inclusions, and both were discarded in 1986 when the FDA updated its Compliance Policy Guidelines on the safety of food additives. Present policy calls for herbal safety to be determined on an *ad hoc* basis, usually following a consumer complaint.[8] There is now no FDA compilation of unsafe or possibly unsafe herbs, but sometimes examples on these older lists are referred to in the literature.

One action that was never taken by members of the herb industry was to prove their products safe and effective and to market them as drugs. The reason for that was money; the costs involved are extremely high. A 1990 report by the Center for the Study of Drug Development at Tufts University placed the average cost for developing a new drug at $231 million and the time involved at 12 years.[9] While these figures might well be double for those required for a traditional herbal remedy, the figures of $115 million and 6 years are still excessive. Such high costs are a particular problem in view of the difficulty of obtaining a patent, and the exclusive marketing rights which it affords, on a traditional drug that may have been used for centuries, even millennia. Unless a novel chemical entity is involved, the likelihood of patent protection is slim, and the capital investment required will never be recovered.

So much for the past. It explains why a simple herb like ginseng can be treated so many different ways in different countries. It also helps us understand why the present situation is such an unsatisfactory one. Those responsible for regulatory affairs do not like it because it is disorderly and presents continuing problems to them. Scientists and clinicians do not like it because they see a number of useful medicines languishing in disuse. Herbal advocates do not like it because they recognize that, if reason is not applied to herbal medicine, then the unreason of paraherbalism will prevail. But most of all, consumers dislike it because they suffer from it in several ways. Their pocketbooks suffer when they pay good money for bad remedies. Still worse, their health suffers because they have difficulty in identifying self-selected remedies that are safe and effective. The lack of sound information and the abundance of misinformation in the herbal field causes normally well-informed critical consumers to become lost in a jungle of exaggerated claims and unsubstantiated assertions.

PROPOSAL FOR REFORM

Establishment of Standards

What needs to be done to address the various herbal regulatory concerns? First of all, it is necessary to establish legal standards of quality for herbs. Since it is obviously impossible to regulate properly something that remains undefined, a first step toward effective control must necessarily be the reestablishment of identity and quality standards of the type that existed when so many of the crude vegetable drugs (herbs) were officially monographed in *The United States Pharmacopeia (USP)* and *The National Formulary (NF)*. A return to official status in these volumes appears unlikely; therefore, it will be necessary to develop some kind of a botanical codex or compendium.

This is not a new idea. In 1977, the Botanical Codex Committee of the American Society of Pharmacognosy recommended that the society undertake the preparation of a volume that would "present in a well-referenced, concise form all information necessary for the identification, determination of purity, uses, and safety of the major botanicals in use today for which no standards have been proposed."[10] It was envisioned that the volume would include some 300 to 400 monographs, and its preparation would be supported financially by commercial organizations, regulatory agencies, and individuals. Although the committee remained active until 1980 and attempted to promote preparation of the volume during that period, funding was not forthcoming, and the project was placed on hold.

Today there appears to be renewed interest in the preparation of such a volume. The necessity of establishing such standards appears to be generally recognized by knowledgeable individuals, and the American Botanical Council also deems its preparation as a necessary first step in the establishment of reputable herbalism. It is hoped that the various interest groups will identify the talent necessary for the preparation of such a volume and will also find a way to fund its publication and distribution.

Another step that must be taken to assure rational herbal regulation and use is the implementation of proper botanical nomenclature to identify a plant source. Because of the imprecision of botanical synonyms and the lack of agreement on the meaning of common names, herbs can be identified properly only by the use of the appropriate Latin binomial. Throughout most of the United States, yellow root (sometimes written yellowroot) is the synonym for *Hydrastis canadensis*, but in some parts of the country, local people identify it with *Xanthorhiza* or even *Coptis* species. When it comes to the identity of snakeroot or mistletoe, the identity of the product is anyone's guess.

Even the Latin binomials change occasionally, as new priorities of nomenclature are established or as taxonomic reclassifications occur. For example, so-called true chamomile flowers were once said to be derived from *Matricaria chamomilla* L. pro parte or from *Chamomilla recutita* L. (Rauschert). More recently, *Matricaria recutita* L. has become the preferred designation.[11] All of these Latin names refer to the identical plant. The herb is also referred to by a wide variety of common names, including Matricaria (once the official *National Formulary* title), true chamomile, German chamomile, Hungarian chamomile, and wild chamomile, among others.

To make matters worse, even the name of the plant family to which this herb belongs has been changed from Compositae to Asteraceae.[12] While it is not incumbent upon those interested in herbs to solve all the complex problems of botanical nomenclature, it is necessary for standard names to be applied to specific plant materials. Uniform, correct botanical nomenclature is prerequisite to the establishment of herbal quality. Publication in 1992 of *Herbs of Commerce*, a listing of the scientific names and preferred synonyms of 550 species, has been very helpful in this regard.[13]

A method permitting certification of the identity and quality of an herb in accordance with appropriate standards is also important. Today, a manufacturer of Aspirin Tablets *USP* must certify, in accordance with legal standards, that they contain not less than 95.0 percent and not more than 105 percent of the labeled amount of $C_9H_8O_4$ (acetylsalicylic acid). And, further, the manufacturer must certify that the $C_9H_8O_4$ meets a whole series of tests ranging from the proper infrared absorption spectrum to the absence of heavy metals. Similar but appropriate standards need to be set for the identity and quality of herbs. Such standards are sorely needed. Numerous reports in the literature detailing cases of atropine poisoning caused by comfrey, nettle, mallow, and burdock (none of which contains atropine) support the difficulty involved in properly identifying herbal materials. There is also the famous case in which clinicians misidentified marihuana as catnip and reported the discovery of a new hallucinogenic smoking material.[14] Certification of identity and quality is the responsibility of the manufacturer (grower) and marketer. In the herbal field, which is comprised of many small operators, such tests would probably need to be conducted for them by qualified commercial laboratories or by a government agency on a fee-for-service basis.

Proving Safety and Efficacy

The next step in the proposed regulatory process is without question the most difficult one. It involves the safety and efficacy of the herbal products and the therapeutic claims that can legally and ethically be made for them. The discussion of this important matter is begun here with the assertion that the various situations that now exist are unsatisfactory, and a uniform policy for at least the technologically advanced nations would be highly desirable.

Proof of safety is the simplest element in this equation and the one most amenable to solution. It can be established relatively easily by appropriate toxicological testing of modest dimension. Besides, most herbs with long-established usage are reasonably safe if employed properly. The few that apparently are not–and these include comfrey, sassafras, coltsfoot, aristolochia, borage, mistletoe, certain types of calamus, and the like–should be withdrawn from the market unless proven to be safe by a would-be distributor.

An entire spectrum of choices opens up when therapeutic claims begin to be discussed. Three of the major options available are:

1. Permit no claims whatsoever, unless substantiated by absolute proof of efficacy obtained in clinical trials carried out according to recognized protocols for new therapeutic agents.
2. Permit reasonable claims to be made, but note that they are based on traditional reputation only and have not been validated by clinical testing.
3. Permit claims, as for any other drug, based on a doctrine of "reasonable certainty," utilizing information gathered from all sources, including reference works, practicing physicians, patients' anecdotal testimony, folkloric sources, etc. Actually, this option is very similar to the practice now prevailing in Canada, which involves accepting herbs and botanicals as drugs on the basis of acknowledged claims and quantitative statements of their active ingredients.

Each of these three regulatory philosophies is actually used in one or more countries today. Let us examine their strengths and weaknesses.

The no-claims policy prevalent in the United States today is satisfactory to no one. It is a continual frustration to the Food and Drug Administration personnel who are put in the position of trying to defend the obvious risk to the consumer on the basis of its relative unimportance. To quote Samuel Page of the FDA Center for Food Safety and Applied Nutrition,[15] the lack of herbal regulation is ". . . an area that regretfully is of economic interest [one-half billion dollars in sales in 1989] but does not do substantial harm."

Page continues, ". . . the agency, with its limited resources, can address [herbs] only if there is suspected direct or indirect health fraud."

A proposal to establish a new category of drugs to be designated "Folklore Medicines" was advanced in Canada by an Expert Advisory Committee on Herbs and Botanical Preparations. Drugs in this category could be marketed with traditional claims of therapeutic efficacy if they had first been demonstrated to be safe. Although the proposal had much to recommend it and seemed reasonable at first glance, it was not adopted in its original form. However, it may be noted parenthetically that, as a result of the study, Canadian officials did decide to allow many commonly used herbs to be sold as drugs with certain limited therapeutic claims.[16] Probably various legal considerations regarding product liability in this litigious age discouraged the authorities from implementing the original proposal. Ensuring the safety of herbal products and at the same time allowing consumers to be properly informed about their traditional use is the regulatory philosophy that prevails today in Britain and France.[17] It has a number of obvious drawbacks.

Perhaps the principal one is that some marketers would be tempted to make outrageous claims about the purported efficacy of their products. If one explores the older herbal literature thoroughly enough, it becomes evident that in many cases a particular herb may have been recommended for a very wide variety of ailments. Although a regulatory body could be established to approve claims for effectiveness, what evidence is that body to use in judging whether the claim is appropriate? Surely it would not allow burdock root to be recommended for the treatment of rabies. Yet Culpeper did just that in his famous herbal, and his recommendation could be construed as a "traditional use."[18] No scientific basis would exist to make a proper judgment on many such claims.

Another drawback to the traditional claims approach is that it provides no incentive for scientists to determine whether an herb is truly useful, thereby discouraging further research and perpetuating the status quo. One has only to compare the volume of research conducted in the field in France and Britain with that in Germany, where the third regulatory philosophy prevails, to recognize the inadequacies of the French-British system.

The third possibility of allowing therapeutic claims based on "reasonable certainty" or "acknowledged claims" seems to me to offer the most promising solution to a very difficult problem. As will be explained in some detail in the next chapter, the German government has established a system of evaluation of phytomedicinals that involves absolute proof of safety and a reasonable certainty of efficacy before such products can be marketed. The conclusions are published in a series of monographs that present, in abbreviated form, the essential data concerning use of the herb. While one might question a few of the recommendations, and while the data on which they are based are not made public, these monographs certainly represent the best collective judgments on phytomedicinal safety and efficacy currently available. Further, the system on which they are based has done much to encourage research in the field of herbal medicine, and many new and significant products have resulted from such activity. Ginkgo biloba extract, echinacea preparations, various chamomile products, milk thistle, and saw palmetto are just a few of the prominent examples.

It might even be appropriate for the FDA to adopt not only the German system of phytomedicinal evaluation but its findings to date as well. The results of such action would not be without precedent because, during the 1980s, nearly 80 percent of the drugs approved for sale in the United States had first been approved in foreign countries.[19] In all of those instances, the FDA did not necessarily rely on foreign data exclusively, but it is obvious that our me-too system of drug approval has done little to encourage innovation. While adoption of the German findings would represent a change in standards of safety and efficacy for botanical drugs, the excellent experience which that advanced nation has had with the system and the nearly total absence of supporting data of American origin would seem to render such an action desirable.

Contrary to the above-stated point of view, some have argued that any special approach to herbal regulation is hypocritical. Moulds and McNeil have noted that ". . . the Australian public expects a high standard of regulations of conventional therapeutic agents, and it is hypocritical to accept a totally different standard for herbal remedies."[20] Although this opinion is understandable, it begs the question.

If we do adhere to the same standards, there will never be any meaningful herbal medicine. Since no one–or no one organization–is going to spend the necessary millions to *prove* herbs effective in the manner required of conventional drugs, it is either necessary to change the rules or to allow the American public to wallow in ignorance. Remember that under our present system, only the name of the herb is allowed to appear on the label. There are no indications of use and no required standards of purity and quality. Such lack of information and quality assurance is definitely detrimental to the health and welfare of the American consumer. Ignorance also encourages quackery, and there is already enough of that in the field. This alternative is unacceptable. Think what conventional medicine would be like today if there had been no herbalism in the past. Extremely important drugs such as the digitalis glycosides and the alkaloids of ergot, cinchona, and opium would be missing from our materia medica. That, too, is a cogent argument for the implementation of a regulatory policy allowing phytomedicinals to be sold following establishment of absolute proof of safety and reasonable certainty of their efficacy.

Besides, different standards already exist for foods, drugs, and related substances. How else can one explain the continued sale of saccharin in the United States when it has been shown to cause cancer in small animals? What about the ongoing marketing of alcoholic beverages and tobacco, both of which have been proven beyond a doubt to be detrimental to the health of the consumer as well as to society in general?

Turning to the drug field, it is only necessary to cite the case of homeopathic remedies that are openly advertised, prescribed, and sold in many countries in spite of the fact that scientific and clinical evidence of their effectiveness is totally lacking. Inverse dose-response relationships of drugs are rare, yet homeopathy attributes that effect to every substance in its materia medica. If all drugs were regulated by one set of standards, homeopathy would have ceased to exist long ago.

It is impossible to deny the need in the United States today for a truly rational system to promote the availability and the rational use of phytomedicinals. With health care costs breaking all records on an almost daily basis and many persons experiencing difficulty in obtaining ready access to the health care system, the use of time-honored plant remedies for many self-limiting ailments could help solve these pressing problems. Unfortunately, under the present restrictions imposed on herbs and herbal labeling in this country, the means of properly utilizing this potentially helpful type of over-the-counter medicament is denied the consumer.

In summary, this proposed solution to the herbal regulatory dilemma is not new. It utilizes several elements that have been proposed previously but for various reasons were never implemented. First, it requires preparation of a botanical codex or similar compendium to establish standards of identity, purity, and quality for all crude vegetable drugs. Second, it mandates that all herbs sold be properly identified by the proper Latin binomial and that a method of determining compliance with the appropriate standards be implemented. Next, it requires that the safety be established of all herbs sold to consumers. Finally, it allows herbs to be sold for the treatment of specified conditions, if their efficacy for those conditions has been proven with reasonable certainty and all other requirements have been met.

This proposal for reform in herbal regulations is not presented as a panacea. It is suggested as the most feasible method of effecting a solution to the present regulatory dilemma. It also would provide a much needed incentive, now sorely lacking, to conduct studies on the safety of the common herbs and on their therapeutic utility as well. It would also assure that only herbs of proven safety be marketed and that the consumer could rely on their effectiveness. Although some may disagree with specific parts of the proposal, there can be no question that its implementation would result in a vast improvement over existing regulatory procedures.

As this is written, the herbal regulatory situation in the United States is a very fluid one, and the outcome is still unknown. The FDA has tentatively adopted a position that would require phytopharmaceuticals to be proven safe and effective by the same costly and unrealistic standards as new chemical entities, or they would have to be withdrawn from the market. The herb-using, cost-conscious public has expressed substantial opposition to this proposed regulation through its elected representatives in the Congress. It is apparent that the final decision will have a considerable influence on the therapeutic use of phytomedicinals in this country for many years to come.

REFERENCE NOTES

1. Duke, J.A. and Ayensu, E.S.: *Medicinal Plants of China*, vol. 1, Reference Publications, Algonac, Michigan, 1985, p. 122.

2. Harlow, D.R.: *Food, Drug, Cosmetic Law Journal* 32:248-274 (1977).

3. Ziporyn, T.: *Journal of the American Medical Association* 254:2037-2046 (1985).

4. Leech, P.N., ed.: *Journal of the American Medical Association* 109:1531-1539 (1937).

5. Davis, A.L., ed.: *Weekly Pharmacy Reports* 11(32):1-4 (1962)

6. Blumenthal, M.: *HerbalGram* No. 23:32-33, 49 (1990).

7. Winter, R.: *A Consumer's Dictionary of Food Additives*, rev. ed., Crown Publishers, Inc., New York, 1984, pp. 8-9.

8. Israelsen, L.: *HerbalGram* 3(3):1-2 (1986).

9. Anon.: *American Pharmacy* NS30(7):10 (1990).

10. Farnsworth, N.R., et al. (7 other authors): *Report of the Botanical Codex Committee*, American Society of Pharmacognosy, Seattle, August 13, 1977, p. 4.

11. Foster, S.: *Chamomile*: Matricaria recutita & Chamaemelum nobile, Botanical Series no. 307, American Botanical Council, Austin, Texas, 1990, 7 pp.

12. Tucker, A.O.: "Botanical Nomenclature of Culinary Herbs and Potherbs," in *Herbs, Spices, and Medicinal Plants: Recent Advances in Botany, Horticulture, and Pharmacology*, vol. 1, L.E. Craker and J.E. Simon, eds., Oryx Press, Phoenix, 1986, pp. 65-67.

13. Foster, S., ed.: *Herbs of Commerce*, American Herbal Products Association, Austin, Texas, 1992, 78 pp.

14. Jackson, B. and Reed, A.: *Journal of the American Medical Association* 207:1349-1350 (1969).

15. Persinos, G., ed.: *Washington Insight* 1(3):1,8 (1988).

16. Blumenthal, M.: *HerbalGram* No. 22:18, 35 (1990).

17. Reuter, H.D.: *Journal of Ethnopharmacology* 32:187-193 (1991).

18. Culpeper, N.: *Culpeper's Complete Herbal*, Richard Evans, London, 1814, p. 36.

19. Abelson, P.H.: *Science* 255:381 (1992).

20. Moulds, R.F.W. and McNeil, J.J.: *The Medical Journal of Australia* 149:572-574 (1989).

Chapter 3

Contents and Use
of the Subsequent Chapters

The herbal monographs found in subsequent chapters do not constitute a comprehensive, encyclopedic listing of all of the more than 300 herbs currently used in Western medicine. Readers who anticipate that approach will not have their expectations realized. The chapters that follow are instead devoted principally to those phytomedicinals that are now considered to be the most useful for treating particular diseases or syndromes. Following brief general discussions of the pathophysiology of the various conditions, monographs of the useful herbs for treating those disorders are arranged in approximate order of their decreasing therapeutic utility. Occasionally, a particular section will contain brief discussions of herbs that are not particularly effective but are nevertheless included because of their popularity. Several minor carminatives in Chapter 4 are a case in point. A very few herbs that are considered totally ineffective or even dangerous to use are included for the same reason. Sarsaparilla and sassafras in Chapter 12 are examples.

Simply because an herb is listed does not mean that it should be used for the particular ailment. For example, phytomedicinals have no place in the self-treatment of self-diagnosed heart disease or cancer. Herbs of potential value in such conditions are discussed to bring them to the attention of professionals who are qualified to use them properly. Hawthorn and taxol are examples. Each monograph must be read carefully to determine the safety, utility, and proper use of the herb discussed there.

Unlike the botanical or alphabetical system utilized in most herbals, the classification of phytomedicines in this volume is based on their principal therapeutic use. Because some of them are useful for more than one condition, they may appear more than once. In most such cases, the minor reference is cross-referenced to the major monograph. Chamomile preparations are, for example, quite useful in the treatment of various kinds of skin conditions. However, since such pharmaceutical preparations are not ordinarily available in the United States, chamomile is merely mentioned under treatments for dermatitis in Chapter 11, and the reader is referred to Chapter 4. There the herb is discussed in detail, principally as a digestive aid, but also with respect to its other beneficial properties.

The contents of the major monographs follow the same general pattern with minor deviations. Ordinarily, the part of the plant used, the scientific name (Latin binomial followed by author citation), and the plant family are presented first, but synonyms, unless they are especially meaningful, are ignored. In a work devoted primarily to the therapeutics of useful herbs, enumeration of the multiplicity of common names was deemed unnecessary, as was much pharmacognostical information such as habitat, production, preservation, marketing, and the like. All of this is readily available elsewhere.

Chemical identification of the active principles (where known) is followed by a discussion of therapeutic use, side effects, dosage and dosage forms, and usually some remarks about the value of the herb in the eyes of an authority such as the United States Food and Drug Administration or Commission E of the German *Bundesgesundheitsamt* (Federal Health Agency), with my additional comments. The FDA and its attitude toward phytomedicinals have been discussed sufficiently in Chapter 2. The activities of Commission E are probably less well-known to American readers, but since they are frequently quoted in the monographs, some explanation of the Commission's role in the evaluation of the safety and efficacy of phytomedicinals is required.

In 1978, the German *Bundesgesundheitsamt* undertook the task of evaluating the safety and efficacy of phytomedicinals. To do this, the agency established a Commission E that was presented with the formidable task of examining appropriate data concerning about 1,400 different herbal drugs corresponding to some 600 to 700 different plant species. The data utilized by the Commission included results obtained from clinical trials, collections of single cases, and scientifically documented medical experience. The latter category comprises both the scientific literature and collective conclusions of medical associations.

Results of the study have been published as Commission E monographs in the *Bundesanzeiger* (Federal Gazette). About 300 such monographs, covering most of the economically important herbal remedies sold in Germany, have appeared to date.[1] Each of these monographs generally provides such information as the identity, composition, use, contraindications, side effects, precautions, dosage, preparations, and effects for those herbs considered effective. For ineffective herbs, comments on the risks involved in consumption and an overall evaluation are substituted for much of the above information.

The Commission E monographs contain the best evaluations of the utility of phytomedicinals currently available. Most experts in the field are in general agreement with the findings reported therein. Occasionally, a different opinion has been expressed. For example, the Commission has found St. John's wort to be an effective, mild antidepressant.[2] Hänsel has noted that convincing, scientifically reliable evidence to support any conclusion that the activity of this herb is comparable to that of the antidepressants presently utilized in therapy is not available.[3] In this volume, the Commission E judgment is therefore tempered somewhat by calling the herb "apparently modestly effective in this regard." Another questionable statement in a Commission E report is the nontherapeutically effective dose of salicin (60-120 mg.) recommended in the monograph on willow bark.[4] Because of some scattered controversial findings of this nature, it is most unfortunate that neither the data used by the Commission in reaching its conclusions nor the minutes of its meetings are available to the public.

Nevertheless, to repeat for emphasis, **the findings of the German Commission E on herb safety and efficacy constitute the most accurate body of scientific knowledge on that subject available in the world today**. They are extensively referred to in this book.

Numerous references are included in the discussions of the various herbs in the following chapters. These will enable any of the principal subjects presented therein to be pursued in additional detail. While it is regretted that many of the key references are written in the German language, this simply reflects the country where most of the investigations have been carried out. The Commission E monographs and the discussion of the various properties of carminatives are just two such examples where comparable information is not available in English. As this is written, English translations of the Commission E monographs are being prepared. A considerable amount of information on herbal use appears for the first time in English in this book.

Some readers may consider it unusual that herbs commonly utilized in traditional Chinese and Indian (Ayurvedic) medicine are not represented more frequently in the subsequent chapters. Many possible entries were considered, but with rare exceptions, such as ephedra, their utility remains unproven by Western scientific standards. The philosophic principles of Chinese and Ayurvedic medicine differ vastly from those on which Western medicine is based and lead, in some cases, to very different conclusions. For example, in this work, Chinese ginseng and American ginseng–different species of the same genus that contain similar active principles–are considered together. As far as can be determined by Western studies, they have similar actions. Yet the Chinese believe they are very different in their properties, the American species being "cold" (yin) and the Oriental being "hot" (yang). In addition, many pharmacological and clinical studies carried out in China and India have lacked adequate "blinding" and controls in their experimental designs; their results are thus very difficult to interpret.

For these reasons, most of the data on which the herbal information in this book is based have been derived from studies in Europe and America. Because of their vast floras, China and India will eventually enrich herbal medicine with remedies of proven value, but to date, their validated contributions have been minimal.

Every effort has been made to be accurate and fair in the presentation of the truly useful herbal remedies. Occasionally, the potential use of a product has been mentioned, but on the whole, the scope of the information has been restricted to statements that are presently substantiated by facts. But in both science and medicine, today's facts may not be the same as tomorrow's. Therefore, as befitting a life-long health professional, I have attempted to present the information in neither a conservative nor a liberal manner, but rather in a conscientious one. It is believed that most readers will appreciate this concept as they peruse the pages that follow.

REFERENCE NOTES

1. Keller, K.: *Journal of Ethnopharmacology* **32**:225-229 (1991).

2. *Bundesanzeiger* (Cologne, Germany): December 5, 1984; January 5, 1989; March 2, 1989.

3. Hänsel, R.: *Phytopharmaka*, 2nd ed., Springer-Verlag, Berlin, 1991, p. 260.

4. *Bundesanzeiger* (Cologne, Germany): December 5, 1984.

Chapter 4

Digestive System Problems

NAUSEA AND VOMITING (MOTION SICKNESS)

Ordinarily preceded by feelings of discomfort and uneasiness, nausea and vomiting are the principal results of motion sickness. These events are controlled by an emetic center in the brain that is influenced by stimuli from peripheral sites, from a so-called chemoreceptor trigger zone (CTZ) in the brain, and/or from the cortex of that organ. Antiemetics usually function by blocking these stimuli. Antihistamines, such as dimenhydrinate for example, prevent peripheral stimuli from reaching the emetic center and are therefore particularly useful in cases of motion sickness or inner ear dysfunction. Anticholinergics, such as scopolamine, are also effective.

However, both of these useful types of drugs are not without unpleasant side effects. Many antihistamines produce drowsiness and subsequently impair mental and physical abilities; the anticholinergics may cause effects ranging from dry mouth and drowsiness to blurred vision and tachycardia. Effective medicines lacking such side effects are considered highly desirable. Although lacking central nervous system (CNS) effects and functioning by a mechanism not well understood, the herbal remedy of choice for preventing motion sickness is:

Ginger

Often mislabeled as a root, ginger is technically a rhizome or underground stem of the plant *Zingiber officinale* Roscoe. Commercial varieties are ordinarily designated according to their geographical origin, such as African ginger, Cochin ginger, or Jamaican ginger. Used in China as a spice and a drug for some 25 centuries, it is now employed throughout the world for both of these purposes, but particularly as a flavoring agent. Its uses in traditional medicine are numerous, but the properties for which it has been most valued are those of a carminative or digestive aid.[1]

More than a decade ago, Mowrey became interested in the antinauseant properties of ginger.[2] Having noted that consumption of ginger-filled capsules prevented him from vomiting during a flu attack, he and Clayson decided to investigate the effects of ginger on motion sickness, a readily controlled producer of nausea. The resulting study, conducted on 36 college students with a high susceptibility to motion sickness, concluded that 940 mg. of powdered ginger was superior to 100 mg. of dimenhydrinate in reducing the symptoms of motion sickness when consumed 20 to 25 minutes prior to tests conducted in a tilted rotating chair.[3]

The results of investigations subsequent to the initial one of Mowrey and Clayson have been quite interesting. An American group consisting of Stott and colleagues reported, in 1984, that ginger had no effect on motion sickness.[4] In 1986, Swedish investigators, Grontved and Hentzer, found ginger significantly better than a placebo in reducing vertigo; it did not have any effect, however, on the nystagmus (oscillation of the eyeballs) of test subjects.[5] Then, Americans led by Wood reported negative results in 1988.[6] They noted that motion sickness is a CNS reaction to vestibular (inner ear) stimulation with only secondary gastrointestinal involvement. Because ginger lacks CNS activity, it was not, they concluded, a useful motion sickness preventive.

More recent European studies have yielded favorable results. Grøntved and colleagues tested the effects of ginger on seasickness in 80 Swedish naval cadets.[7] They concluded that ginger reduced vomiting and cold sweating. Also, fewer symptoms of nausea and vertigo were reported, but there is a question about the statistical significance of these observations.

In Germany, Holtmann and colleagues carried out tests to determine the mechanism of ginger's positive effects.[8] They concluded that the drug does not influence the inner ear or the oculomotor system, both of which are of primary importance in motion sickness. Thus, a CNS effect of ginger should be ruled out, and it must be concluded that the antiemetic mechanism of action of ginger is of a gastrointestinal nature.

To summarize, it is interesting to note that, after the initial studies of ginger's favorable effects on motion sickness by an American team, five additional investigations have been made to date. Two were conducted in the United States with negative results; the three made in Europe all had positive outcomes. Analysis of some of the findings previously mentioned, together with other nonpublished data, has been sufficient to convince Commission E of the German Federal Health Agency that ginger is effective not only for indigestion but also in preventing the symptoms of motion sickness. They so recommend it at an average daily dose level of 2 to 4 g.[9]

Whatever activity ginger possesses may be attributed to a contained volatile oil (1-3 percent) responsible for its characteristic odor, and an oleoresin (mixture of volatile oil and resin) responsible for its pungency. The principal components of the volatile oil are the sesquiterpene hydrocarbons zingiberene and bisabolene, which are accompanied by a number of other hydrocarbons and alcohols. Nonvolatile pungent components include the shogaols and the gingerols.[10]

In small animals, these pungent components have been shown to exhibit a large number of effects including cardiotonic, antipyretic, analgesic, antitussive, and sedative properties;[11] however, their significance in human medicine has not been demonstrated. There are numerous references in both the medical and popular press suggesting that ginger is useful in preventing or treating a variety of human ailments including migraine headache, elevated cholesterol levels, rheumatism, hepatotoxicity, burns, peptic ulcers, depression, aging penile vascular changes, and impotence. Evidence supporting such claims is, as yet, insubstantial. The herb does have a long-standing and apparently valid reputation as a digestive aid.

There are also reports that ginger is useful in the treatment of nausea of all kinds, not just that associated with motion sickness. A recent study has shown ginger to be as effective as metoclopramide in reducing the incidence of nausea and vomiting in a group of 60 women following major gynecological surgery.[12] It should be noted that the investigation was carried out in Britain, not in the United States. The predominately negative results obtained with ginger as an antinauseant in this country may possibly be attributed to use of a poor quality product.

Backon has noted that ginger inhibits thromboxane synthetase and acts as a prostacyclin agonist. Thus it could prolong bleeding time and produce immunological changes. In view of this, he suggests caution in using ginger to treat postoperative nausea.[13] However, no toxic or unpleasant side effects have been reported from the consumption of ginger in therapeutic amounts for the prevention of motion sickness. In addition to receiving approval of the German Commission E as previously noted, the herb appears on the GRAS list of the U.S. Food and Drug Administration.

Ginger is ordinarily taken in the form of hard gelatin capsules, each containing 500 mg. of the powdered rhizome. To prevent motion sickness, swallow 2 capsules 30 minutes before departure and then 1 to 2 more as symptoms begin to occur, probably about every 4 hours. A pleasant way to consume the product is in the form of the candied or crystallized ginger that is readily available in Oriental food markets. This is prepared by boiling the fresh rhizome in a syrup solution, and the resulting product is marketed in slices sprinkled with granulated sugar. A piece 1 inch square and 0.25-inch (25 mm. square × 6 mm.) thick weighs about 4 g. Because of the loss of some active principles during preparation and the presence of more water in this type of ginger, such a piece is probably equivalent to about one 500 mg. capsule.

APPETITE LOSS

It has long been believed that the consumption of bitter herbs stimulates the appetite. When a bitter substance interacts with the taste buds at the base of the tongue, stimuli pass, primarily by way of the glossopharyngeal nerve, to a group of special cells in the cerebral cortex. The taste is interpreted there as bitter, and this causes stimuli to be forwarded through the vagus nerve to both the salivary glands and the stomach. The flow of both saliva and gastric juice is increased, as is the motility of the stomach. This stimulation of the digestive process enhances the appetite. Additional augmentation occurs when the bitter-tasting material actually reaches the stomach and promotes the secretion of gastrin, a hormone that intensifies the secretion of hydrochloric acid by the gastric glands.[14]

Two theories exist regarding the effectiveness of bitter substances as appetite stimulants; there is scanty experimental evidence supporting either.[15] The first holds that the stimulation of digestion by the administration of bitters to normal persons is greater than that induced by regular foods. The second postulates that such increases occur only in persons suffering from secretory deficiencies, but in normal persons, no increased digestive capability is induced. Additional studies are required to determine the precise degree of utility of bitter herbs as appetite stimulants and digestion promoters in normal persons.

Nevertheless, the use of "bitter tonics" is widespread in Europe, where they are often consumed in the form of strong (about 40 percent) alcoholic extracts. Because alcohol is also a known appetite stimulant based on both its local irritating and CNS effects, it becomes difficult to separate its action from that of the contained bitter herbs. The use of bitter drugs to stimulate appetite is not rational in those cases of chronic appetite losses that are manifestations of more severe conditions such as anorexia nervosa. It may be useful, however, in treating loss of appetite in elderly persons suffering from reduced production of stomach acid and digestive enzymes.

Significant Bitter Herbs

Gentian

One of the most popular of the bitter tonic herbs is gentian. It represents the dried rhizome and roots (underground parts) of *Gentiana lutea* L. (Gentianaceae), a moderately tall perennial herb with clusters of characteristic orange-yellow flowers. The best quality product is dried quickly and retains its white color. Slow-dried gentian becomes reddish in color and develops a distinctive aroma but contains less of the desired bitter principles. However, even the well-prepared herb darkens and develops the distinctive odor after a period of 6 to 8 months.[16] The useful constituents of gentian are secoiridoid glycosides, principally gentiopicroside (gentiopicrin), swertiamarin, and especially amarogentin, which are primarily responsible for its bitter taste. Amarogentin, which occurs in gentian in a concentration of 0.05 percent, surpasses the bitter value of the more abundant gentiopicroside by a factor of 5,000. These principles are accompanied by a number of xanthones, alkaloids, phenolic acids, characteristic sugars, such as the bitter gentiobiose, etc.

The bitter taste of gentian is probably best known to most Americans in the form of Angostura Bitters, a proprietary cocktail flavoring that contains gentian, not angostura. Other vestiges in this country of the numerous varieties of highly alcoholic stomach bitters that were once sold to stimulate the appetite and facilitate digestion are the bitter aperitifs such as Campari and vermouth. However, the former relies on quinine for its bitterness and the latter on a complex mixture of herbal ingredients that varies with the producer but always includes wormwood. Wormwood is GRAS-listed in the United States and may be used here as a flavor only if it is free of thujone, a toxic bicyclic terpene. In Europe, gentian aperitifs and liqueurs are both numerous and popular. It must be noted, however, that gentian schnapps is a beverage distilled from fermented gentian rhizomes and roots; consequently, it does not contain the nonvolatile bitter principles.

The traditional use of gentian as an appetite stimulant in some malnourished individuals, especially the elderly, is probably valid. German Commission E has reported that the bitter principles in gentian stimulate the taste buds and increase by reflex action the flow of saliva and stomach secretions. For this reason, it is said to act as a tonic.[17] While animal studies have shown that gentian and its constituents may be potentially useful in the treatment of stomach ulcers,[18] that, as well as numerous other reported uses, requires verification.

The herb is probably best consumed in the form of a decoction prepared by gently boiling 1/2 level teaspoonful (ca. 1g.) of coarsely powdered root in one-half cup (120 ml.) of water for 5 minutes. Strain and drink while still warm about 30 minutes before mealtime. If the beverage thus prepared is so strong as to be unpleasant, reduce the amount of herb accordingly. Consumption of gentian may be repeated up to a total of 4 times daily. The herb may cause headache in certain predisposed individuals.

Centaury

Another member of the Gentianaceae that is very similar to gentian in its constituents and effects is centaury. This herb consists of the dried aboveground parts–leaves, stems, and flowers–of *Centaurium erythraea* Rafn., a plant native to Europe and Asia but naturalized in the United States. Like gentian, it contains amarogentin, gentiopicroside, swertiamarin, and a number of related bitter principles. It is used for precisely the same purpose as gentian, but Pahlow recommends that 1 heaping teaspoonful (ca. 2 g.) of the herb be extracted with a cup (240 ml.) of *cold* water for 6 to 10 hours, stirring occasionally, to prepare the most active beverage.[19] This "tea" should be warmed before drinking. The herb is approved by German Commission E for treatment of appetite loss and indigestion.[20]

Minor Bitter Herbs

Other, less important bitter herbs that may be encountered from time to time include:

Bitterstick. This consists of the dried plant, *Swertia chirata* Buch.-Ham., family Gentianaceae.

Blessed Thistle. This is the dried aboveground plant, *Cnicus benedictus* L., (*Carbenia benedicta* Adans), family Asteraceae.

Bogbean. The herb comprises the dried leaves of *Menyanthes trifoliata* L., family Menyanthaceae.

None has any particular advantage over gentian or centaury, and they will not be discussed further here. Another bitter herb, but one that cannot be recommended because of its potential toxicity, is:

Wormwood. The dried leaves and flowering tops of *Artemisia absinthium* L. (family Asteraceae) were mentioned briefly as a constituent in vermouth. The herb will not be considered in detail because the volatile oil,, which it yields to the extent of 0.2 to 0.8 percent, contains variable amounts (35 percent is not uncommon) of a toxic mixture of (–)-thujone and (+)-isothujone. Even though Wichtl has maintained that relatively little thujone is found in aqueous wormwood preparations (teas),[21] it does not seem prudent to employ a potentially poisonous herb as a bitter when other, safer ones are available.

CONSTIPATION

Herbs in this category were formerly classified on their relative potency based on the amount of cramping they produced and the relative consistency of the stool. *Laxatives* designated the mildest category; *cathartics* were stronger; and *drastic purgatives*, the most formidable. Now, the products are usually organized according to their mode of action.

Bulk-producing herbs are those which, when consumed with sufficient liquid, expand in volume, thereby stimulating peristalsis and emptying of the bowel. They are probably the safest laxatives, functioning as they do in a fashion identical to high-residue foods; in consequence, they are rather widely used.[22]

A large number of herbs function as *stimulants*, due primarily to their content of anthraquinones. These do increase the motility of the colon, but what is even more important, they induce changes in its surface cells, promoting the accumulation of water and electrolytes.[23] Drawbacks to the use of such drugs include their tendency to promote over-emptying and reduction of spontaneous bowel function, thus leading to development of the so-called laxative habit. Being absorbed into the general circulation, anthraquinones find their way not only into the bile, urine, and saliva, but also into the milk of lactating women. Because the identity and content of active principles and the resultant activities of these drugs vary greatly, each must be considered individually.

Bulk-Producing Laxatives

Plantago Seed

Probably the most popular of these laxatives, plantago seed is also known as psyllium seed. This herb is official in *The United*

States Pharmacopeia XXII where it is described as the cleaned, dried, ripe seed of *Plantago psyllium* L. or of *Plantago indica* L., known in commerce as Spanish or French Psyllium Seed; or of *Plantago ovata* Forskal, known in commerce as Blond Psyllium or Indian Plantago Seed. All of these plants are members of the family Plantaginaceae.

The seed coats or husks of plantago seeds contain cells that are filled with mucilage that is neither absorbed nor digested in the intestinal tract. In contact with water it swells to a large volume, thus providing both bulk and lubrication, causing either the whole seed or the husks to act as an effective bulk-producing laxative. Obviously, it is necessary to drink large amounts of water when taking this herb.[24] The usual dose of the seed is 7.5 g. (2 heaping teaspoonfuls); one teaspoonful of the husks will provide the same effect. Plantago seed husks, usually referred to as psyllium in the health food industry, are readily available both prepackaged and in bulk. For best results, stir the husks into a glass of water, juice, or milk and drink it quickly before the mixture has a chance to thicken.

In recent years, some studies have shown that plantago seed, like other higher fiber products, lowers cholesterol levels in the blood of humans. German health authorities have found both plantago seed and husks safe and effective for this purpose,[25] but neither has been approved for such use in the United States. In 1989, two psyllium-containing breakfast cereals with the names Benefit and Healthwise appeared on the market. Benefit has now been withdrawn, but as of this writing, Healthwise is still generally available.[26] It has recently been relabeled to indicate that a very small percentage of people may develop allergic reactions when exposed to psyllium. Nevertheless, the product was banned from sale in the state of Texas where a federal district judge in Dallas declared the cereal to be a drug, not a food.[27] This is an excellent example of the difficulty that sometimes exists in distinguishing between a drug and a food. Without question, a few botanicals are both. Although it is widely sold as an OTC drug, there appears to be no valid reason to prohibit the sale of plantago seed as a healthful food as well.

Stimulant Laxatives

Significant Stimulant Laxatives

Cascara Sagrada

Of all the herbs that function as stimulants, the best is certainly cascara sagrada. This herb enjoys official status in *The United States Pharmacopeia XXII* where it is described as the dried bark of *Rhamnus purshiana* DC. (family Rhamnaceae). Obtained from a small tree native to the Pacific Northwest, the bark should be collected at least one year prior to use in order to allow some of the harsh laxative constituents, i.e., the reduced emodin glycosides (anthrones) originally present in the bark, to be oxidized naturally to less active monomeric forms. Cascara owes its action to a mixture of active principles consisting largely of cascarosides A, B, C, and D, with other anthraquinone glycosides in minor amounts. Bark of *USP* quality contains not less than 7 percent total hydroxyanthracene derivatives calculated as cascaroside A on a dried basis. The cascarosides should make up at least 60 percent of this total.

Cascara is probably the mildest of the anthraquinone stimulant laxatives, producing only minor effects on the small intestine. Because of its relatively mild action, the herb is the least likely of the stimulant laxatives to produce undesirable side effects such as griping or dependence. Nevertheless, the active principles are excreted in mother's milk, so nursing mothers, and for that matter, pregnant women, should avoid taking it or other anthraquinone-containing herbs.

Although cascara is normally taken in the form of prepared pharmaceutical dosage forms such as an extract, fluidextract, or aromatic fluidextract, it is also possible to consume the powdered bark in capsule form. Average dose is 1 g. (about 1/2 teaspoonful). Cascara tea is not popular because of its extremely bitter taste. The herb is an ingredient in several popular over-the-counter (OTC) laxatives.[28]

Buckthorn (Frangula) Bark

This product is very similar to cascara, being obtained from its near-relative *Rhamnus frangula* L. (family Rhamnaceae), a shrub or small tree that grows in Europe and western Asia. Its laxative effect is due to the presence of anthraquinone derivatives, particularly glucofrangulin A and B and frangulin A and B. Like cascara, buckthorn bark should be aged one year prior to use in order to allow the reduced glycosides (anthrones) with their harsh laxative action to be converted to milder oxidized forms.[29]

Properly aged buckthorn bark is also comparable to cascara in its relatively gentle laxative action. In spite of this, it is not commonly used in the United States where it is overshadowed by the more popular native species *Rhamnus purshiana*. It is a very popular drug in its native Europe. Cascara is somewhat less expensive than buckthorn bark in this country, so there appears to be no particular advantage in using the latter.

The German Commission E has found buckthorn bark to be an effective stimulating laxative.[30] Average dose is 1 g. A fluidextract of the botanical, once official in the *NF*, remains a useful dosage form.

Senna

Probably the most widely used of the anthraquinone-containing stimulant laxatives is senna. Official in the *USP XXII*, senna is described there as consisting of the dried leaflet of *Cassia acutifolia* Delile, known in commerce as Alexandria Senna, or of *Cassia angustifolia* Vahl, known in commerce as Tinnevelly Senna. These low-growing shrubs of the family Fabaceae are native to Egypt or to the Middle East and India, respectively. Some taxonomists now group both of these species together under a single scientific name, *Senna alexandrina* Mill. Dianthrone glycosides, particularly sennosides A, A_1, B, C, D, and G, together with various other anthraquinone derivates, account for the laxative action of senna.[23] The total complex of senna glycosides is also official in the *USP* under the title Sennosides.

Although senna is not as mild in its action as cascara, producing more smooth muscle contractions with attendant cramping, it is nevertheless more widely used because it is considerably cheaper. Bulk lots of the herb are only about one-half the price of cascara. A fluidextract and a syrup made from the leaflets are available, as are tablets prepared from a mixture of the purified active ingredients–

so-called sennosides. A bitter-tasting tea can be prepared from 0.5 to 2 g. (ca.1/2-1 teaspoonful) of the herb. Some prefer a beverage prepared by soaking the leaflets in cold water for 10 to 12 hours and then straining. Such a preparation will be more active than the customary hot tea and will contain less resinous material.[31]

Other Stimulant Laxatives

Other laxative herbs in this category that are encountered with some frequency include:

Aloe (Aloes). Also official in the *USP XXII*, the drug consists of the dried latex of several species of *Aloë*, especially *A. barbadensis* Mill. (*A. vera* L.), known in commerce as Curaçao aloe, or of *A. ferox* Mill., and hybrids of these species with *A. africana* Mill. and *A. spicata* Bak., known in commerce as Cape aloe. All of these species are members of the family Liliaceae. The anthraquinone glycosides aloin A and B (formerly designated barbaloin) render aloe an extremely potent laxative. Although still widely used abroad, its use in the United States has declined in recent years, rendering it of relatively minor therapeutic significance.

Aloe is obtained from specialized cells known as pericyclic tubules that occur at the border of the outer and inner cortical layers of the mesophyll located just beneath the epidermis of the leaves of the aloe plant. The bitter yellow latex found there is drained and dried to a reddish-black glistening mass. This drug is totally different from the colorless mucilaginous gel (aloe gel or aloe vera gel) obtained from the parenchyma tissue making up the central portion of the aloe leaf. Aloe gel is primarily a wound-healing agent and is discussed in Chapter 11; it should never be confused with aloe, the laxative.

Rhubarb. This consists of the dried rhizome and root of *Rheum officinale* Baill. or *R. palmatum* L. or of related species or of hybrids grown in China (Chinese rhubarb); or of *R. emodi* Wall. or *R. webbianum* Royle native to India, Pakistan, or Nepal (Indian rhubarb). It is not common garden rhubarb, *R.* x *cultorum* Hort. (*R. rhaponticum* L.), which is relatively inactive.

As is the case with aloe, this laxative herb is much more potent than cascara or senna. Its use almost always causes intestinal griping or colic. For this reason, rhubarb is seldom employed as a laxative today and cannot be considered an herb of choice. A very popular "tonic" preparation, widely sold in Europe and occasionally marketed in this country, is *Swedish Bitters*. Its active constituents include senna, aloe, and rhubarb; frequent use is not recommended.[32]

Minor Laxative Herbs

There are many other laxative herbs. Some, such as colocynth, jalap, and podophyllum, are drastic purgatives; others, such as dandelion root and manna, are so mild as to be uncertain in their action. None provides any advantage over plantago seed, cascara, buckthorn bark, or senna.

DIARRHEA

Diarrhea is characterized by increased fluidity and volume of the stool, almost always accompanied by increased frequency of bowel movement. Although normal functioning of the bowels varies greatly in different individuals, and this must be taken into account in the definition, diarrhea ordinarily involves defecation more than three times daily. The condition may be acute or chronic, and the causes are numerous, ranging from allergies to viral infections. Self-limited episodes of less than 48 hours duration are very common; they are usually attributed to intestinal infections caused by various organisms such as *Escherichia coli* or enterovirus.

Such conditions are often treated with nonspecific antidiarrheal agents of plant origin. The most effective of these is opium, usually employed in the form of a camphorated tincture known as paregoric. However, since this drug is a controlled substance and available only on the prescription of a physician, other herbal remedies are much more widely used. Their effectiveness is due to their content of the polyphenolic substances popularly known as tannins.

These compounds tend to arrest diarrhea by their astringent action, which reduces intestinal inflammation. They effect this by binding to the surface protein layer of the inflamed mucous membranes, causing it to thicken, thereby hindering resorption of toxic materials and restricting secretions. Tannins which are most effective are those that are slowly released from the various complexes in which they exist in the plant after reaching the lower gastrointestinal tract.[33] This prevents stomach upset and also allows the tannin to act at the site where it is most effective. The most widely used astringent herbs are obtained from several edible berry plants.

Because of their similarities, the leaves of three plants may be considered as a group:

Blackberry Leaves–the dried leaves of *Rubus fruticosus* L. (family Rosaceae);

Blueberry Leaves–the dried leaves of *Vaccinium corymbosum* L. or *V. myrtillus* L. (family Ericaceae); and

Raspberry Leaves–the dried leaves of *Rubus idaeus* L. or of *R. strigosus* Michx. (family Rosaceae).

All of the leaves contain appreciable amounts of tannin; quantities up to 10 percent have been reported for blueberry leaves[34] and a range of 8 percent to possibly 14 percent for blackberry leaves.[35] All three are consumed in the form of teas, usually prepared by pouring one cup (240 ml.) of boiling water over 1 to 2 teaspoons (ca. 2-4 g.) of the finely cut leaves and steeping for 10 to 15 minutes. Alternatively, the plant material may be macerated in cold water for about 2 hours and then strained to yield the beverage. A cup of the tea may be drunk up to 6 times a day as necessary to control the diarrhea. However, if the condition lasts more than 2 or 3 days, it is obviously not amenable to treatment with astringent herbs.

The teas from all three berry leaves may also be used effectively as a mouthwash or gargle for sore mouth and inflammation of the mucous membranes of the throat.

Raspberry leaf tea has a persistent traditional reputation of utility in treating a wide variety of female conditions ranging from diabetes and menstrual difficulties to those associated with pregnancy, such as morning sickness and labor pains. One reputable scientific reference[36] continues to note that the tea has been a traditional remedy for "painful and profuse menstruation and for use before and during confinement." The German Commission E concluded that the leaf has not been proven effective for any of these complaints.[37] See Chapter 9 for additional details.

Other useful antidiarrheal herbs include the following.

Blackberry Root

Also known by the Latin title *rubus*, this was listed in *The National Formulary* until 1936, where it was defined as the dried bark from the rhizome and roots of plants of the section *Eubatus* Focke of the genus *Rubus* L. (family Rosaceae). The section *Eubatus* includes more than 50 species and cultivated varieties of the plants commonly referred to as blackberries and dewberries. It is of little value to enumerate them here, since they are all similar qualitatively and quantitatively in their tannin content and are used similarly.

Although it appears on the GRAS list, the root bark no longer seems to be a common article of commerce in the United States. It may be self-collected and dried, in which case it is best used by extracting the finely powdered or cut bark in boiling water for 20 minutes since the tannins are more difficult to extract from bark than from leaf material. Blackberry root bark is an effective anti-diarrheal agent, but the traditional use of the root as a preventative treatment for dropsy is unproven; it cannot be recommended for this latter purpose.[38]

Blueberries

Dried blueberry fruits (*Vaccinium corymbosum* L. in the United States and *V. myrtillus* L. in Europe) are highly recommended, particularly by European authorities, to combat simple diarrhea. They do not appear to be an item of commerce in this country but may be prepared by drying fresh berries in the sun. Do not use the fresh blueberries themselves for treatment of diarrhea. They may even exert a laxative effect.[34]

Use of the dried berries involves chewing 3 tablespoonfuls (30 g.) and swallowing them. Alternatively, a drink may be prepared by boiling the crushed fruits in water for about 10 minutes, then straining and drinking. In addition to tannins, the berries contain pectin which, by virtue of its adsorbent properties, is also useful in the treatment of diarrhea.

There are several other reputed uses of these fruits, particularly of *V. myrtillus* which are often referred to in the American herbal literature as **Bilberries**. Preliminary studies indicate that a concentrated extract of anthocyanosides obtained from these berries may benefit visual acuity as well as provide protection against macular degeneration, glaucoma, cataracts, and the like.[39] It must be emphasized that these claims are based on studies carried out primarily in small animals or on small numbers of human subjects. Extensive clinical studies in human beings are required to verify these initial findings before the herb can be recommended for these purposes. Dried bilberries nevertheless remain a useful treatment for diarrhea. In the meantime, a bilberry extract containing 25 percent anthocyanosides calculated as anthocyanidin is widely sold as a phytomedicine in Europe, and it is available in this country as a food supplement.

INDIGESTION–DYSPEPSIA

In modern medicine, digestive disturbances are treated with a variety of drugs ranging from antacids and H_2-receptor antagonists in the case of acid peptic disorders to synthetic antispasmodics for functional bowel complaints and cramps. In herbal medicine, stomach upsets, bloating, and related digestive problems are customarily treated with certain plant drugs, usually those containing volatile oils, that act as carminatives. Narrowly defined, a carminative is an agent that relieves flatus (gas in the stomach or intestine). But present-day usage attributes a much broader range of action to such drugs.

Carminatives

According to Schilcher,[40] carminative effects on the stomach, gall bladder, and intestinal tract result from at least five different activities, the intensity of each of which varies, depending on the identity of the specific herb. These effects are:

1. Local stimulation of the stomach lining, leading initially to an increase in tonus and an intensification of rhythmic contractions facilitating the eructation (belching) of air from that organ; this is promoted by relaxation of the lower esophageal sphincter.

2. Reflexive increase in stomach secretions resulting in improved digestion.
3. Antispasmodic or spasmolytic effects on smooth muscle; the intestine is especially relaxed, facilitating the passage of intestinal gas.
4. Antiseptic action, limiting the development of undesirable microorganisms.
5. Promotion of bile flow (cholagogue effect), facilitating digestion and absorption of nutrients.

Determination of the effectiveness of volatile-oil-containing herbs in treating gastrointestinal problems is difficult, and the results are controversial. In a series of in-vitro experiments, Forster and colleagues concluded that the antispasmodic activities of the most effective plant extracts tested–including peppermint, chamomile, and caraway–were less than those produced by atropine.[41] Hof-Mussler has noted that observations of the effects of carminative herbs on isolated smooth muscle preparations have not necessarily been confirmed by subsequent in-vivo experiments.[42] Clinical studies of the spasmolytic action of volatile oils have yielded mixed results. To be effective, relatively high concentrations are required at the site of action. There is little doubt that, in many cases, the observed activity of these herbs in alleviating indigestion is due in part, but not entirely, to the placebo effect. There is also little question that they are effective, at least subjectively. Persons with gastric distress do feel better after consuming them. For that reason, they continue to be used to reduce such discomfort.

The mode of consumption is of considerable importance. In this country, teas are the most common dosage forms. But volatile oils are relatively insoluble in water, so teas are not very efficient therapeutic agents. For example, it has been estimated that chamomile tea contains only about 10 to 15 percent of the volatile oil present in the plant material.[43] Fluidextracts or tinctures of the herbs prepared with 30 to 70 percent alcohol are much more effective, but they are not always available commercially and must be self-prepared. Alcoholic solutions of the purified volatile oils are also employed for the same purpose.

Significant Carminative Herbs

Peppermint

Although many plant materials contain volatile oils and therefore possess some carminative properties, one of the most effective and widely used is certainly peppermint. Consisting of the leaves and flowering tops of *Mentha* x *piperita* L. (family Lamiaceae), this herb is officially listed in the *NF XVII*. It contains 0.5 to 4 percent (average, about 1.5 percent) of a volatile oil that is composed of 50 to 78 percent free (–)-menthol and from 5 to 20 percent menthol combined in various esters such as the acetate or isovalerate. It also contains (+)- and (–)-menthone, (+)-isomenthone, (+)-neomenthone, (+)-menthofuran, and eucalyptol, as well as other monoterpenes.[44] Although flavonoid pigments found in the leaf may also exert some physiological effects,[45] there is little question that most of the activity is due to the constituents of the oil, primarily menthol.

Peppermint oil has long been an extremely popular flavoring agent in products ranging from chewing gum to after-dinner mints. It is probably the most widely used carminative, acting in the broad sense defined by Schilcher.[40] The German Commission E has found peppermint or its volatile oil to be effective as a spasmolytic (particularly useful for discomfort caused by spasms in the upper digestive tract), a stimulant of the flow of bile, an antibacterial, and a promoter of gastric secretions.[46] On the other hand, in 1990, the United States Food and Drug Administration declared peppermint oil to be ineffective as a digestive aid and banned its use as a nonprescription drug for this purpose in this country.[47] What this actually means is that the FDA was not presented with evidence proving the efficacy of peppermint as a digestive aid. As previously explained, this would not be financially feasible in this country. It does not mean that peppermint oil is an ineffective aid to digestion.

Peppermint is GRAS-listed, and both it and peppermint oil are recognized as flavoring agents in the *NF XVII*. Peppermint tea is prepared by pouring about 2/3 cup (160 ml.) of boiling water over 1 tablespoonful (1.5 g.) of the recently dried leaves and steeping for 5 to 10 minutes. Drink this amount of tea 3 to 4 times daily between meals to relieve upset stomach. Peppermint Spirit (*USP XXII*), an alcoholic solution containing 10 percent peppermint oil and 1 percent peppermint leaf extract, is also available in pharmacies. The usual dose is 1 ml. (20 drops) taken with water.

Regular consumption of peppermint tea is considered safe for normal persons, although excessive use of the volatile oil (0.3 g. = 12 drops) may produce some toxic effects.[48] Allergic reactions to menthol have also been reported.[45] Considerable caution should be observed in giving peppermint tea to infants or very small children since they may experience an unpleasant choking sensation due to the contained menthol.[49]

Chamomile

Another extremely popular herb for the treatment of indigestion, as well as various other conditions, is chamomile. German or Hungarian chamomile, often referred to as true chamomile or matricaria, consists of the dried flower heads of a plant now technically designated *Matricaria recutita* L. In the older literature on medicinal plants, it is usually referred to as *Matricaria chamomilla* L.p.p. or as *Chamomilla recutita* (L.) Rauschert. At least seven other scientific names have been used to designate the plant. It is a member of the daisy family, formerly known as the Compositae, but is now called the Asteraceae by most taxonomists. The important thing to remember when attempting to maneuver through this nomenclatural maze of five English common names, ten scientific names, and two plant family designations is that all of the names refer to a single species of plant. Its popularity as a traditional medicine is so great that in Germany it was declared the medicinal plant of the year for 1987.[50]

A related plant is Roman or English chamomile, composed of the flower heads of *Chamaemelum nobile* (L.) All. (family Asteraceae). Its constituents are not identical to those of German chamomile, but both plants are similarly employed. In Britain, Roman chamomile is the herb of choice; on the continent, German chamomile is preferred. The latter is also the species most commonly consumed in the United States.

The literature on the chamomiles is extensive. *Die Kamille*, a 152-page book by H. Schilcher, provides comprehensive coverage.[51] Mann and Staba's 1986 review is the most recent one in the English language.[52] It provides 220 references to various agronomic, botanical, chemical, and pharmacological aspects of the herbs.

A blue-colored volatile oil, obtained from the chamomiles by steam distillation or solvent extraction in yields up to nearly 2 percent, contains the principal anti-inflammatory and antispasmodic constituents of the plants. These include, in the case of German chamomile, the terpenoids (–)-α-bisabolol, (–)-α-bisabololoxides A and B, and matricin. In addition, certain flavonoids, such as apigenin and apigenin-7-glucoside, are also present in the flower heads themselves and certainly add to the herb's antispasmodic activity.

The chamomiles are used internally for digestive disturbances. Like peppermint, they possess carminative (antispasmodic) effects, but unlike peppermint, they exert, in addition, a pronounced anti-inflammatory activity on the gastrointestinal tract. In this country, chamomile tea is most widely used for this purpose. It is prepared by pouring boiling water over 1 heaping tablespoonful (about 3 g.) of the flower heads and allowing them to steep in a covered vessel for 10 to 15 minutes. A cup of freshly prepared tea is drunk between meals 3 or 4 times daily for stomach or intestinal disturbances. As previously noted, only a small fraction of the volatile oil is extracted in this way, but the flavonoids are present, and there is reason to believe the tea provides a cumulative beneficial effect.

Both German and Roman chamomile are considered safe for normal human consumption, being GRAS-listed by the FDA. Some allergies have been reported, therefore persons with known sensitivities to them or to various other members of the Asteraceae (e.g., ragweed, asters, chrysanthemums) should be cautious about consuming chamomile teas. However, this rather remote possibility has been greatly overemphasized in some of the nonmedical literature.[53] Only five cases of allergy specifically attributed to German chamomile were identified worldwide between 1887 and 1982.[54] The German Commission E considers German chamomile effective internally for gastrointestinal (GI) spasm and inflammatory conditions of the GI tract. It was also found to be effective when used as a mouthwash for irritations and minor infections of the mouth and gums.

In Europe today, a large number of pharmaceutical preparations are available containing either extracts of chamomile or chamomile volatile oil. Some are creams or lotions intended to treat various skin irritations, including those caused by bacterial infections. Other forms are suitable for inhalation and are designed to relieve bronchial irritation; still others are used as baths or rinses to alleviate irritations in the anogenital regions. Commission E has concluded that German chamomile is also effective for these purposes.[55] However, since none of these preparations have been approved for use as an OTC drug in the United States, and such dosage forms are not ordinarily available here, their therapeutic use will not be discussed further.

Finally, it should be noted that chamomile herb is not inexpensive and is relatively easy to adulterate. To assure quality, purchase it only in the form of the whole flower heads, which are easy to identify with a little experience, and make certain that no appreciable quantity of stems is present (less than 10 percent). It is best to avoid pulverized or powdered chamomile, the quality of which is difficult to determine, even for experts. Any preparations containing chamomile oil (most will be foreign-made) should be acquired only from firms having outstanding reputations for quality products. Three-quarters of the commercial chamomile oil samples examined in 1987 were found to be adulterated, often with cheaper, synthetically prepared, blue-colored compounds such as guaiazulene.[56]

Minor Carminative Herbs

Other herbs frequently used as digestive aids for the carminative properties of their contained volatile oils include:

Anise. This is the dried ripe fruit of *Pimpinella anisum* L., family Apiaceae. The fruit is commonly referred to in the popular literature as a seed.

Caraway. This herb consists of the dried ripe fruit (often called the seed) of *Carum carvi* L., family Apiaceae.

Coriander. This herb is composed of the dried ripe fruit (often called the seed) of *Coriandrum sativum* L., family Apiaceae. Two varieties of this species are commonly employed: var. *vulgare* Alef. and var. *microcarpum* DC.

Fennel. This is the dried ripe fruit (often called the seed) of various cultivated varieties of *Foeniculum vulgare* Mill., family Apiaceae.

All of the above are GRAS-listed, and all four of them were found to be effective treatments for indigestion by the German Commission E.[57] However, all have relatively weak activities and offer no particular advantage over either peppermint or chamomile as digestive aids, except in the uncommon case of an allergy to one of these latter herbs. Each of the herbs is administered in the form of a tea prepared by pouring 1 cup (240 ml.) of boiling water over 1 teaspoonful (2.5 g.) of the crushed fruit, steeping for 10 to 15 minutes, and straining prior to drinking.

An herb that has been used for centuries to relieve digestive disorders but which cannot be recommended on the basis of present-day knowledge is:

Calamus. The aromatic rhizome (underground stem) of *Acorus calamus* L., family Araceae, comprises this drug. At least four subtypes of this plant exist, two of which contain large amounts of β-asarone (*cis*-isoasarone), a compound found in experiments to promote the development of malignant tumors in the intestines of rats. A third type of calamus contains much lesser amounts of this toxic compound, and a fourth (drug type 1), native to North America, is β-asarone free. However, these types are not normally differentiated in commerce; consequently, the use of calamus and its extracts is prohibited in the United States.[58]

Cholagogues

Pain of obscure origin in the upper portion of the stomach, frequently intensified by the consumption of fatty foods and accompanied by a feeling of fullness or bloating, is often attributed to an inadequate flow of bile from the liver. Traditionally, dyspepsia of this sort has been treated with herbal cholagogues–that is, agents acting either to empty the gallbladder (cholekinetics) or to stimulate the production of bile (choleretics), or both.

Hänsel has noted that many clinicians consider the use of such agents obsolete, and the terms themselves are not utilized in modern gastroenterology. Nevertheless, cholagogue phytomedicinals are widely used and do provide relief from this type of indigestion.

They may also play some role in the prevention of gallstone formation, although evidence in support of this effect is less convincing.[59]

Herbs previously mentioned in this chapter that also function as useful cholagogues include gentian and peppermint. Although horehound possesses choleretic properties, its principal use is as an expectorant, so it is discussed in Chapter 6. As is the case with some other herbs in this category, the activity of these three plants in promoting bile flow is relatively mild, and they are considered to be both safe and effective.

Turmeric

Of the remaining herbal cholagogues, perhaps the best known and most widely used is turmeric. Consisting of the rhizome of *Curcuma domestica* Val. (synonym *C. longa* L.) of the family Zingiberaceae, turmeric has long been used as a yellow food coloring and spice. It is one of the principal ingredients in curry powder. Related species, such as *C. zanthorrhiza* Roxb. (Javanese yellow root) and *C. zedoaria* (Christm.) Rosc. (commonly known as zedoary) have similar, but quantitatively different, therapeutic properties due to different concentrations of identical or closely related constituents.

In addition to 4.2 to 14 percent of an essential oil consisting of about 60 percent of sesquiterpene ketones known as turmerones, turmeric contains three major curcuminoids, of which curcumin (diferuloylmethane) is the most significant.[60] These curcuminoids are responsible for the yellow color of the herb.

The choleretic action of turmeric and related species is attributed primarily to its volatile oil; the cholekinetic effects, as well as appreciable anti-inflammatory properties, are believed to be due to the curcuminoids.[61] Animal studies have also demonstrated a hepatoprotective effect for turmeric, but evidence to support its use in cases of liver disease in humans is not yet available.

Curcumin is not well absorbed following oral administration; only traces subsequently appear in the blood when turmeric is given by mouth. However, the compound is active at relatively low concentrations, and it may also produce a local action in the gastrointestinal tract. The relatively poor absorption of the curcuminoids would seem to emphasize the role of the volatile oil constituents in the activity of turmeric.

Regardless of the identity of its active constituents, turmeric is a widely used and apparently effective cholagogue and digestive aid. Both it and Javanese yellow root have been declared effective for such use by the German Commission E.[62] Because both the contained volatile oil and the curcuminoids are relatively water insoluble, teas for therapeutic purposes are seldom made from turmeric.[63] Instead, hydroalcoholic fluidextracts or tinctures of the herb or encapsulated powders are the dosage forms customarily employed. The usual dose is 1.5 to 3.0 g. of turmeric daily; preparations are consumed in equivalent quantities. Use over an extended period of time infrequently results in gastric disturbances. Persons suffering from gallstones or blockage of the bile duct should avoid consuming turmeric or even curry powder (28 percent turmeric).

Boldo

The dried leaves of *Peumus boldus* Mol. (family Monimiaceae), an evergreen shrub native to Chile, have an ancient reputation as a "hepatic tonic," diuretic, and laxative. The herb contains about 2 percent of a volatile oil, the principal constituents of which are ascaridole, eucalyptol, and p-cymol. About 0.25 to 0.5 percent of an alkaloidal mixture is also present. Boldine, an aporphine alkaloid, constitutes about one-fourth of the total; the remainder consists of about 16 different alkaloids.[59] Boldine is responsible for both the choleretic and diuretic activity of the leaves.[64] Although the herb may increase the flow of urine substantially, the mechanism of action is still unknown, so it is uncertain if boldine's action is one of true diuresis or simply aquaresis, as is the case with most herbs in this category. See Chapter 5 for further discussion of urinary tract problems.

Although Commission E has approved the use of boldo for the treatment of dyspepsia as well as for stomach and intestinal cramps, it must be noted that the volatile oil in the leaves contains about 40 percent ascaridole, a rather toxic component. Since no chronic toxicity testing has been carried out, Hänsel has recommended that prolonged use of the herb or any consumption by pregnant women be avoided. Boldo is normally taken as a tea prepared from 1 to 2 teaspoonfuls (1.5-3 g.) of the herb. The average choleretic dose is 3 g. daily.[65]

Dandelion

The dried rhizome and roots of *Taraxacum officinale* Weber (family Asteraceae) is mentioned here primarily as a matter of record. Otherwise, some readers might believe this common herb, usually known as dandelion root, had been overlooked. Scientific evidence to support claims of any significant effects for this centuries-old home remedy is simply insufficient to allow it to be considered as useful.

Dandelion root apparently possesses very mild choleretic properties, and the leaf is thought to be a feeble diuretic (aquaretic). However, most of the animal and clinical investigations on which these claims are based date from the 1930s.[66] The root, together with the overground parts of the plant, is said by the German Commission E to have choleretic, diuretic, and appetite stimulating properties,[67] but additional verification is required. Some authorities believe that the use of dandelion root as a choleretic stems principally from the fact that the plant has a yellow flower and, according to the Doctrine of Signatures, would be a useful remedy for jaundice. The plant lacks any significant documented pharmacological activity.[68]

HEPATOTOXICITY (LIVER DAMAGE)

Medical treatment of liver damage or potential damage resulting from certain disease states or the consumption of hepatotoxins is largely symptomatic and supportive. Agents such as thioctic acid have been used experimentally in the treatment of deadly amanita mushroom poisoning, but the reported results are variable. Likewise, the value of corticosteroids in treating such conditions as alcoholic hepatitis is uncertain.

Milk Thistle

There is at least one herbal remedy that has shown considerable promise as a liver protectant in conditions of this sort. The one that has been widely used and extensively investigated as a cure or preventive for a wide range of liver problems is milk thistle. This herb consists of the ripe fruits, freed from their pappus (tuft of silky hairs), of *Silybum marianum* (L.) Gaertn. (family Asteraceae). A crude mixture of antihepatotoxic principles was first isolated from the plant and designated silymarin. It is contained in the fruit in concentrations ranging from 1 to 4 percent. Subsequently, silymarin was shown to consist of a large number of flavonolignans, including principally silybin accompanied by isosilybin, dehydrosilybin, silydianin, silychristin, and possibly several others, depending on the variety examined.[69]

Studies in small animals have shown conclusively that silymarin exerts a liver protective effect against a variety of toxins including those of the deadly amanita.[70] Human trials have also been encouraging for conditions including hepatitis and cirrhosis of various origins.[71] The results of numerous studies suggest that silymarin has considerable therapeutic potential, protecting intact liver cells or cells not yet irreversibly damaged by acting on the cell membranes to prevent the entry of toxic substances. Protein synthesis is also stimulated, thereby accelerating the regeneration process and the production of hepatocytes (liver parenchyma cells). The biochemical mechanism by which this increased protein synthesis is achieved has been established.[72] In addition, silymarin functions as a free-radical scavenger and antioxidant.[73]

The German Commission E endorses use of the herb as a supportive treatment for chronic inflammatory liver conditions and cirrhosis. Average daily dose is 12 to 15 g.[74] This is equivalent to about 200 to 400 mg. of silymarin. Unfortunately, silymarin is very poorly soluble in water, so the herb is not effective in the form of a tea. Studies show that such a beverage contains less than 10 percent of the initial activity in the plant material.[75] Coupled with the fact that silymarin is relatively poorly absorbed (20-50 percent) from the GI tract, it is obvious that the administration of concentrated products is advantageous. Milk thistle is marketed in this country in the form of capsules, usually containing 200 mg. each of a concentrated extract representing 140 mg. of silymarin. Toxic effects resulting from the consumption of milk thistle have apparently not been reported.

The only other liver protective herb that need be mentioned at all, and then only briefly, follows.

Schizandra

Also spelled schisandra, this herb consists of the dried ripe fruits of *Schisandra chinensis* (Turcz.) Baill. (family Schisandraceae). The fruits and seeds of this plant, native to China, have been extensively investigated chemically and found to contain more than 30 different lignans, including schizandrin, wuweizisu C, and gomisins A, B, C, D, F, and G. Some of these compounds have been studied in small animals for physiological activity. Several of them appear to protect the liver from toxic substances. Even though a number of schizandra products or combinations are currently marketed, their safety and efficacy for any purpose, particularly antihepatotoxic effects, remain unproven.[76] The consumption of schizandra cannot now be recommended.

GASTRIC AND DUODENAL (PEPTIC) ULCERS

Treatment of peptic ulcers is normally aimed at neutralizing hydrochloric acid by the frequent administration of antacids or by decreasing the secretory activity of the stomach. This latter objective is now usually achieved by the administration of histamine H_2-receptor antagonists (cimetidine, rantidine), although the older anticholinergic drugs (belladonna alkaloids) are still occasionally employed. Treatment should be intensive, and during its course, the intake of irritants, such as aspirin, other nonsteroidal anti-inflammatory agents, or alcohol, must be strictly avoided.

Effective herbal treatments for ulcers are not numerous. Aside from belladonna, which due to the potential toxicity of its alkaloidal constituents is a prescription drug and unavailable for self-treatment, possibly the only truly effective plant remedy is described below.

Licorice

Also known as glycyrrhiza, this herb consists of the dried rhizome (underground stem) and roots of *Glycyrrhiza glabra* L., known in commerce as Spanish licorice, or of *G. glabra* L. var. *glandulifera* (Wald. & Kit.) Reg. & Herd., known in commerce as Russian licorice, or of other varieties of *G. glabra* L. that yield a yellow and sweet wood (family Fabaceae). It is often referred to as licorice root.

During World War II, a Dutch physician named F. E. Revers noted that peptic ulcer patients improved markedly when treated with a paste containing 40 percent licorice extract prepared by a local pharmacist in the small city of Heerenveen in the northern part of the Netherlands.[77] Revers used licorice paste to treat successfully a number of ulcer patients, but in doing so noted a serious side effect. About 20 percent of the patients developed edema, principally in the face and extremities. However, those unpleasant effects disappeared promptly and completely when treatment was discontinued.

During the intervening half century, a great many studies have been conducted on licorice, its constituents, and their effects. Much has been learned about the therapeutic usefulness and the side effects of the herb, but in essence, the findings remain the same. Licorice is useful in the treatment of peptic ulcers; depending on the dose, it may produce serious side effects. These undesirable effects are mineralocorticoid in nature. Specifically, they include headache, lethargy, sodium and water retention (the edema noted by Revers), excessive excretion of potassium, and high blood pressure. Eventually, heart failure or cardiac arrest may result. The medical literature is replete with references to cases of poisoning produced by over-consumption of licorice candy or licorice-containing tobacco.[78]

Glycyrrhizin (glycyrrhizic acid), a triterpene glycoside with saponinlike properties, is contained in licorice in a range of 2 to 14 percent. Plant material of good quality contains at least 4 percent. It is responsible for the sweet taste of the herb, being some 50 times sweeter than sugar. The glycoside has pronounced expectorant and antitussive properties.[79] On hydrolysis, glycyrrhizin loses its sweet taste and is converted to glycyrrhetinic acid (glycyrrhetic acid) and two molecules of glucuronic acid. Both glycyrrhizin and its triterpene aglycone, glycyrrhetinic acid, possess distinct anti-inflammatory and antiallergic properties. These account for licorice's effectiveness in treating ulcers. Both compounds also possess mineralocorticoid activity; that accounts for the herb's side effects.

Recent studies have shown that the mechanism involved in producing both the beneficial and the deleterious effects is similar. Glycyrrhetinic acid inhibits 15-hydroxyprostaglandin dehydrogenase and Δ^{13}-prostaglandin reductase, two enzymes important in the metabolism of prostaglandins E and $F_{2\alpha}$. This inhibition promotes the healing of peptic ulcers because of increased levels of prostaglandins in the stomach are cytoprotective to the gastric mucosa. The acid also inhibits another enzyme, 11β-hydroxysteroid dehydrogenase, thus increasing the glucocorticoid concentration in mineralocorticoid-responsive tissues, which causes sodium retention, potassium excretion, and high blood pressure. Structural studies of both types of enzymes indicate a sufficient similarity to postulate derivation from a common precursor.[80] Thus, these two actions of licorice are almost certainly inseparable.

Carbenoxolone, a semisynthetic derivative of glycyrrhetinic acid, is widely marketed outside the United States as an antiulcer drug. It is not yet available in this country so persons wishing to utilize licorice for treatment of this condition are restricted to the herb itself. Normally, it is consumed in the form of a beverage prepared by adding about 1/2 cup (120 ml.) of boiling water to 1 teaspoonful (2-4 g.) of the herb and simmering the mixture for 5 minutes. After cooling, strain and drink this quantity of beverage 3 times daily after meals. The German Commission E has approved the use of licorice in ulcer therapy but cautions that the treatment should not be continued longer than 4 to 6 weeks.[81] It recommends a dosage level of 200 to 600 mg. of glycyrrhizin daily; with average quality herb, the above regimen would provide an amount about midpoint in that range. Elderly persons or those suffering from cardiovascular disease, liver or kidney problems, or potassium deficiency should avoid consuming licorice unless they do so while under the care of a physician.

Licorice also has a considerable reputation as an expectorant and cough suppressant, being frequently utilized in the treatment of symptoms associated with the common cold. Lozenges and candies containing licorice extract are especially suitable, but particularly in the United States, one must make certain that they do contain real licorice. Most "licorice" candy manufactured in this country is simply flavored with anise oil.

In addition to licorice's antiulcer and expectorant/cough suppressant activities, a number of other potential uses have been studied in small animals and, in some cases, in human beings.[82] As a result, the herb is postulated to possess hypolipidemic (cholesterol and triglyceride lowering), anticariogenic (antiplaque and anti-tooth decay), antimicrobial and antiviral, immunosuppressive, antianemia, and antihepatotoxic properties. Adequate evidence is not available to support the effectiveness of licorice in any of these conditions, but its local application as a hydrocortisone potentiator in preparations used to treat various skin conditions seems to hold considerable promise.[83]

Ginger

Investigations in small animals have shown that extracts of fresh ginger (see discussion on "Nausea and Vomiting" in this chapter) inhibited gastric secretion and the formation of stress-induced lesions.[84] The antiulcer activity of the herb requires confirmation but is certainly worthy of further study.

REFERENCE NOTES

1. Tyler, V.E.: *The Honest Herbal*, 3rd ed., Pharmaceutical Products Press, New York, 1993, pp. 147-148.

2. Mowrey, D.B.: *The Scientific Validation of Herbal Medicine*, Keats Publishing, New Canaan, Connecticut, 1986, p. 198.

3. Mowrey, D.B. and Clayson, D. .: *Lancet* I: 655-657 (1982).

4. Stott, J.R.R., Hubble, M.P., and Spencer, M.B.: *Advisory Group for Aerospace Research and Development. Conference Proceedings 372* **39**:1-6 (1984).

5. Grøntved, A. and Hentzer, E.: *ORL* **48**:282-286 (1986).

6. Wood, C.D., Manno, J.E., Wood, M.J., Manno, B.R., and Mims, M.E.: *Clinical Research Practices and Drug Regulatory Affairs* **6**:129-136 (1988).

7. Grøntved, A., Brask, T., Kambskard, J., and Hentzer, E.: *Acta Oto-Laryngologica* (Stockholm) **105**:45-49 (1988).

8. Holtmann, S., Clarke, A. H., Scherer, H., and Höhn, M.: *Acta Oto-Laryngologica* (Stockholm) **108**:168-174 (1989).

9. *Bundesanzeiger* (Cologne, Germany): May 5, 1988.

10. Awang, D.V.C: *Canadian Pharmaceutical Journal* **125**:309-311 (1992).

11. *Lawrence Review of Natural Products*: April, 1986.

12. Bone, M.E., Wilkinson, D.J., Young, J.R., McNeil, J., and Charlton, S.: *Anaesthesia* 45:669-671 (1990).

13. Backon, J.: *Anaesthesia*, 46:705-706 (1991).

14. Haas, H.: *Arzneipflanzenkunde*, B.I. Wissenschaftsverlag, Mannheim, 1991, p. 78.

15. Hänsel, R.: *Phytopharmaka*, 2nd ed., Springer-Verlag, Berlin, 1991, pp. 121-123.

16. List, P.H. and Hörhammer, L., eds.: *Hagers Handbuch der Pharmazeutischen Praxis*, 4th ed., vol. 4, Springer-Verlag, Berlin, 1973, pp. 1115.

17. *Bundesanzeiger* (Cologne, Germany): November 30, 1985; March 6, 1990.

18. Tanaka, S., Furukawa, T., Adachi, K., and Ishimoto, M.: *Iryo* 42:591-595 (1988).

19. Pahlow, M.: *Das grosse Buch der Heilpflanzen*, Gräfe und Unzer, Munich, 1985, pp. 330-331.

20. *Bundesanzeiger* (Cologne, Germany): July 6, 1988; March 6, 1990.

21. Wichtl, M., ed.: *Teedrogen*, Wissenschaftliche Verlagsgesellschaft, Stuttgart, 1984, pp. 363-365.

22. Brunton, L.L.: "Chapter 38" in *Goodman and Gilman's The Pharmacological Basis of Therapeutics*, 8th ed., A.L. Gilman et al., eds., Pergamon Press, New York, 1990, pp. 914-932.

23. Jekat, F. W., Winterhoff, H., and Kemper, F.H.: *Zeitschrift für Phytotherapie* 11:177-184 (1990).

24. Tyler, V.E., Brady, L.R., and Robbers, J.E.: *Pharmacognosy*, 9th ed., Lea & Febiger, Philadelphia, 1988, pp. 52-53.

25. *Bundesanzeiger* (Cologne, Germany): February 1, 1990.

26. Geslewitz, G.: *Health Foods Business* 36(10):58-59 (1990).

27. Anon.: *American Herb Association Quarterly Newsletter* 7(4):9 (1991).

28. Tyler, V.E., Brady, L.R., and Robbers, J.E.: *Pharmacognosy*, 9th ed., Lea & Febinger, Philadelphia, 1988, pp. 60-62.

29. Wichtl, M., ed.: *Teedrogen*, Wissenschaftliche Verlagsgesellschaft, Stuttgart, 1984, pp. 113-115.

30. *Bundesanzeiger* (Cologne, Germany): December 5, 1984.

31. Wichtl, M., ed.: *Teedrogen*, Wissenschaftliche Verlagsgesellschaft, Stuttgart, 1984, pp. 311-314.

32. Beck, H. and Beck, K.: *Schaufenster* (supplement to *Deutsche Apotheker Zeitung*) 31(8/9):33-34 (1982).

33. Hänsel, R. and Haas, T.: *Therapie mit Phytopharmaka*, rev. ed., Springer-Verlag, Berlin, 1984, pp. 137-140.

34. Frohne, D.: *Zeitschrift für Phytotherapie* 11:209-213 (1990).

35. Wichtl, M., ed.: *Teedrogen*, Wissenschaftliche Verlagsgesellschaft, Stuttgart, 1984, pp. 89-90.

36. Reynolds, J.E.F., ed.: *Martindale: The Extra Pharmacopoeia*, 29th ed., The Pharmaceutical Press, London, 1989, p. 1609.

37. *Bundesanzeiger* (Cologne, Germany): August 14, 1987.

38. *Bundesanzeiger* (Cologne, Germany): February 1, 1990.

39. Murray, M.T.: *The Healing Power of Herbs*, Prima Publishing, Rocklin, California, 1992, pp. 223-230.

40. Schilcher, H.: *Deutsche Apotheker Zeitung* **124**:1433-1442 (1984).

41. Forster, H.B., Niklas, H., and Lutz, S.: *Planta Medica* **40**:309-319 (1980).

42. Hof-Mussler, S.: *Deutsche Apotheker Zeitung* **130**:2407-2410 (1990).

43. Tyler, V.E., Brady, L.R., and Robbers, J.E.: *Pharmacognosy*, 9th ed., Lea & Febiger, Philadelphia, 1988, pp. 466-467.

44. Ibid., p. 116.

45. *Lawrence Review of Natural Products:* July, 1990.

46. *Bundesanzeiger* (Cologne, Germany): November 30, 1985; March 13, 1986.

47. Blumenthal, M.: *HerbalGram* No. 23:32-33, 49 (1990).

48. Wichtl, M.: *Deutsche Apotheker Zeitung* **123**:2114 (1983).

49. Pahlow, M.: *Das grosse Buch der Heilpflanzen*, Gräfe und Unzer, Munich, 1985, pp. 258-260.

50. Carle, R. and Isaac, O.: *Zeitschrift für Phytotherapie* **8**:67-77 (1987).

51. Schilcher, H.: *Die Kamille*, Wissenschaftliche Verlagsgesellschaft, Stuttgart, 1987, 152 pp.

52. Mann, C. and Staba, J.: "The Chemistry, Pharmacology, and Commercial Formulations of Chamomile," in *Herbs, Spices, and Medicinal Plants: Recent Advances in Botany, Horticulture, and Pharmacology*, vol. 1, L.E. Craker and J.E. Simon, eds., Oryx Press, Phoenix, Arizona, 1986, pp. 233-280.

53. Lewis, W.H.: *Economic Botany* **46**:426-430 (1992).

54. Hausen, B.M., Busker, E., and Carle, R.: *Planta Medica* **50**:229-234 (1984).

55. *Bundesanzeiger* (Cologne, Germany): December 5, 1984.

56. Carle, R., Fleischhauer, I., and Fehr, D.: *Deutsche Apotheker Zeitung* **127**:2451-2457 (1987).

57. *Bundesanzeiger* (Cologne, Germany): July 6, 1988; February 1, 1990; November 30, 1985; April 19, 1991.

58. *Lawrence Review of Natural Products:* July, 1989.

59. Hänsel, R.: *Phytopharmaka*, 2nd ed., Springer-Verlag, Berlin, 1991, pp. 186-191.

60. Ammon, H.P.T. and Wahl, M.A.: *Planta Medica* **57**:1-7 (1991).

61. Jaspersen-Schib, R.: *Schweize Apotheker-Zeitung* **129**:706-710 (1991).

62. *Bundesanzeiger* (Cologne, Germany): November 30, 1985.

63. Wichtl, M., ed.: *Teedrogen*, Wissenschaftliche Verlagsgesellschaft, Stuttgart, 1984, pp. 205-206.

64. *Lawrence Review of Natural Products:* May, 1991.

65. *Bundesanzeiger* (Cologne, Germany): April 23, 1987.

66. Wichtl, M., ed.: *Teedrogen*, Wissenschaftliche Verlagsgesellschaft, Stuttgart, 1984, pp. 217-219.

67. *Bundesanzeiger* (Cologne, Germany): December 5, 1984.

68. *Lawrence Review of Natural Products:* December, 1987.

69. Wagner, H. and Seligmann, O.: "Liver Therapeutic Drugs from *Silybum marianum,*" in *Advances in Chinese Medicinal Materials Research,* H.M. Chang, H.W. Yeung, W.-W. Tso, and A. Koo, eds., World Scientific Publishing, Singapore, 1985, pp. 247-256.

70. *Lawrence Review of Natural Products:* March, 1988.

71. Ferenci, P. et al. (8 other authors): *Journal of Hepatology* **9**:105-113 (1989).

72. Sonnenbichler, J. and Zetl, I.: *Planta Medica* **58** (Suppl.):A580 (1992).

73. Leng-Peschlow, E. and Strenge-Hesse, A.: *Zeitschrift für Phytotherapie* **12**:162-174 (1991).

74. *Bundesanzeiger* (Cologne, Germany): March 13, 1986.

75. Merfort, I. and Willuhn, G.: *Deutsche Apotheker Zeitung* **125**:695-696 (1985).

76. *Lawrence Review of Natural Products:* June, 1988.

77. Nieman, C.: *Chemist and Druggist* **177**.741-745 (1962).

78. Tyler, V.E.: *The Honest Herbal,* 3rd ed., Pharmaceutical Products Press, Binghamton, New York, 1993, pp. 197-199.

79. Chandler, R.F.: *Canadian Pharmaceutical Journal* **118**:420-424 (1985).

80. Baker, M.E. and Fanestil, D.D.: *Lancet* **337**:428-429 (1991).

81. *Bundesanzeiger* (Cologne, Germany): May 15, 1986.

82. Wren, R.C.: *Potter's New Cyclopaedia of Botanical Drugs and Preparations,* C.W. Daniel, Saffron Waldon, England, 1988, pp. 173-175.

83. Teelucksingh, S., Mackie, A.D.R., Burt, D., McIntyre, M.A., Brett, L., and Edwards, C.R.W.: *Lancet* **335**:1060-1063 (1990).

84. Sertie, J.A.A., Basile, A.C., Oshiro, T.T., Silva, F.D., and Mazella, A.A.G.: *Fitoterapia* **63**:55-59 (1992).

Chapter 5

Kidney, Urinary Tract, and Prostate Problems

INFECTIONS AND KIDNEY STONES

The kidneys function to remove waste from the body while preserving the chemical integrity of its cells and tissues. They work to maintain an appropriate concentration of electrolytes, amino acids, and glucose, as well as foreign substances, in the plasma and lymph. Although diuretics are commonly thought of as increasing the volume of urine excreted, they actually do much more than that.

There are now several types of widely used synthetic diuretics. These differ markedly in their exact site and mode of action, but basically, all are used to treat various kinds of edema by enhancing both fluid and electrolyte excretion, thereby reducing the amount of extracellular fluid. Many of the beneficial effects of such diuretics, including the control of hypertension, derive not merely from their ability to stimulate the elimination of water but of the electrolytes Na^+, Cl^-, and HCO_3^- as well.[1]

Technically, the classic herbal diuretic drugs are not diuretics at all but are more accurately designated aquaretics. Usually containing volatile oils, flavonoids, saponins, and/or tannins, they function to increase the volume of urine by promoting blood flow in the kidneys, thereby raising the glomerular filtration rate.[2] However, unlike the synthetic diuretics, they do not retard the resorption of Na^+ and Cl^- in the renal tubules, so quantities of these electrolytes are retained in the body and not excreted along with the water. This means that the herbal aquaretics are not suited for the treatment of edema and especially not for hypertension.[3]

Nevertheless, these herbs can prove useful for certain other conditions–for example, minor infections–that are benefited by an increased volume of urine. According to Schilcher, these include pyelonephritis (local infection of the renal tissues), urethritis or ureteritis (inflammation of the urethra or of a ureter), cystitis (inflammation of the urinary bladder), and the like. An increased urine flow is helpful in the prevention of kidney stones.[4] Some of the herbs also exhibit antibacterial properties which, in combination with the increased urinary output, are useful in combating infection. Consequently, phytomedicinals with aquaretic and/or antiseptic properties will be considered here in the same category. In addition, one plant product is included primarily for its antiseptic properties and another, not for either of these effects, but because it prevents infection.

Significant Aquaretic-Antiseptic Herbs

Goldenrod

Probably the most effective and safest of these is goldenrod. Although its value is scarcely recognized in this country, the above-ground parts of several species of *Solidago* are widely used in Europe to treat inflammations of the urinary tract and to prevent the formation, or facilitate elimination, of kidney stones. In Europe, *S. virgaurea* L., as well as *S. serotina* Ait., *S. canadensis* L., and their hybrids, are all used more or less interchangeably.

The genus *Solidago* of the family Asteraceae is notorious for its ability to hybridize, much to the consternation of botanists who recognize about 130 species in the United States.[5] Deam collected 27 species in Indiana alone.[6] Although there are some qualitative and quantitative differences in their anti-inflammatory and bacteriostatic properties, the aquaretic properties of all those goldenrods that have been investigated are similar enough to permit them to be grouped together.[7] The information that follows is based largely on studies conducted on the European goldenrod (*S. virgaurea*).

Goldenrod contains a number of saponins based on polygalic acid; at least 12 diterpenes; phenolic glycosides, especially leiocarposide; and various miscellaneous flavonoids, tannins, polysaccharides, and the like.[8] The plant's aquaretic action is sometimes attributed to the flavonoids, but an isolated flavonoid mixture proved relatively inactive in animal studies.[7] Saponins may enhance their effects. The glycoside leiocarposide has been shown to have both anti-inflammatory and analgesic properties in tests carried out in rats.[9] These effects are probably due to the fact that the glycoside is hydrolyzed in the intestinal tract–although very slowly and incompletely–to salicylic acid.[10] In spite of this relative metabolic stability of leiocarposide, Polish investigators noted that it had significant diuretic activity in rats.[11] Interestingly, they also found that the diuretic effect of the glycoside was reduced by the presence of flavonoids and/or saponins. The exact identity of the constituents responsible for the aquaretic effects of goldenrod thus remains somewhat controversial, although most authors continue to ascribe it to the contained mixture of flavonoids and saponins.[12]

As is the case with almost all herbs, preliminary studies of goldenrod have reported other activities, including antifungal properties in the triterpene saponin fraction[13] and antitumor activity in the polysaccharides.[14] These are merely initial indications and have, as yet, no therapeutic utility.

In spite of some uncertainty regarding the nature of its active principles, a decoction of goldenrod is an effective aquaretic. It is prepared by adding 1 to 2 teaspoonfuls (3-5 g.) of the dried herb to 1/2 pint (240 ml.) of water, bringing it to a boil, and allowing it to stand for 2 minutes before straining and drinking.[15] The usual dose ranges from 0.2 to 0.4 ounces (6-12 g.) of the herb per day.[16]

German Commission E has endorsed the herb as a diuretic, anti-inflammatory, and mild antispasmodic. Toxicity and contraindications are not reported. In this regard, it is superior to most other aquaretics of plant origin.

Parsley

All parts of the plant, *Petroselinum crispum* (Mill.) Nym. of the family Apiaceae, contain varying amounts of a volatile oil with aquaretic activity; about 0.1 percent of the oil is found in the root, 0.3 percent in the leaf, and 2 to 7 percent in the fruit.[17] The aquaretic effect is attributed to the presence of two major components, myristicin and apiol. Concentrations of these constituents vary depending on the variety of parsley from which the oil is obtained. However, some may contain 60 to 80 percent apiol, others 50 to 60 percent myristicin.

In addition to their aquaretic properties, both apiol and myristicin act as uterine stimulants, and the former was once widely used as an abortifacient drug. The oil also contains appreciable amounts of furocoumarins or psoralens, compounds that cause photosensitivity on exposure to sunlight. Because of the presence in the volatile oil of these uterine-stimulant and photosensitizing constituents, use of the oil-rich seeds, or the isolated oil itself, with their greater potential for toxicity is not recommended. The German Commission E does recommend the leaves and roots of parsley as aquaretics to reduce urinary tract inflammation and to facilitate the passage of kidney stones. Average daily dose is 6 g.[18] Many times this amount is consumed by persons who enjoy the Lebanese salad tabbouleh.

Nevertheless, for pregnant women and those light-skinned persons who may be subject to phototoxic effects, the consumption of parsley, either as a nutrient or for therapeutic purposes, is best avoided. As is the case with other volatile-oil-containing aquaretics, parsley functions as an irritant to the epithelial tissues of the kidney, thus increasing the blood flow and glomerular filtration rate. For this reason, it should be used with considerable caution by those suffering from kidney disease.

Juniper

The most active but also the most potentially toxic of the volatile-oil-containing aquaretic/antiseptic herbs consists of the dried ripe fruits (berries) of *Juniperus communis* L. and its variety *depressa* Pursh of the family Cupressaceae. Quality fruits normally yield 1 to 2 percent of a volatile oil that contains various terpene hydrocarbons, especially α- and β-pinenes; sesquiterpenes, such as carophyllene and cadinene; and its principal aquaretic, the terpene alcohol terpinen-4-ol.[19]

Both juniper berries and their steam-distilled oil have ancient reputations as diuretics and genitourinary antiseptics, and were official in the first edition of the *USP* in 1820.[20] However, it was gradually recognized that, as a result of its irritant action, the drug caused injurious effects to the kidneys. It was deleted from the official compendia in 1960.[21] Although the herb is recommended by German Commission E for the treatment of indigestion, it is not approved as a single-ingredient aquaretic.[22]

The exact composition of juniper oil is quite variable. Schilcher has theorized that oils containing a low ratio (e.g., 3:1) of the irritating terpene hydrocarbons to the nonirritating, active aquaretic terpinen-4-ol do not exhibit nephrotoxicity. However, some oils have a hydrocarbon to alcohol ratio as high as 55:1 and are prone to cause kidney damage characterized by albuminuria or renal hematuria.[7] This hypothesis requires additional pharmacological testing.

Because there is no simple way for the potential consumer to measure the terpene hydrocarbon to alcohol ratio in the oil contained in juniper berries, the only sensible alternative is not to use the herb as a therapeutic agent. The very small amounts of the oil used to flavor gin are certainly no more harmful than the beverage alcohol itself.

Minor Aquaretic Herbs

There are two minor herbal aquaretics that require at least a brief mention. Although not as effective as the plants previously discussed and relatively little used in the United States, they are common and modestly effective ingredients in many of the diuretic teas sold in Europe and have a long tradition of folkloric use there.

Birch Leaves

These consist of the dried leaves of the silver or white birch, *Betula verrucosa* Erh. or *B. pubescens* Erh., family Betulaceae. They contain 2 to 3 percent of flavonoids, especially hyperoside and quercitrin, as well as various proanthocyanidins. Up to 0.5 percent of ascorbic acid and a trace of volatile oil are also present.[23]

Aqueous and alcoholic extracts of the leaves produced significant aquaresis in rats, an activity attributed to their flavonoid content.[24] The German Commission E has endorsed the use of birch leaves as a drug that produces increased urinary output and is of value in treating kidney and urinary tract infections.[25] Toxicity and contraindications have not been reported. An adequate intake of water by the patient is a necessity during such treatment.

Lovage Root

The dried root of *Levisticum officinale* W. D. J. Koch, family Apiaceae, also possesses mild aquaretic properties. A heavy volatile oil occurs in the root, usually in amounts ranging from 0.6 to 1.0 percent. Up to 70 percent of the oil consists of alkylphthalides. While these constituents are responsible for the characteristic odor of the oil, they play a limited role, if any, in its aquaretic activity.[26] This effect is due mainly to the terpene derivatives in the oil.

Small animal tests of lovage's aquaretic action have produced extremely variable results. In humans, its activity is probably less than that of juniper but greater than that produced by birch leaves. One of the alkylphthalides present in the oil, ligustilide, possesses antispasmodic properties. The German Commission E recognizes the efficacy of lovage root as an aquaretic for the treatment of urinary tract inflammation and the prevention of kidney stones.[27] Recommended daily dose is 4 to 8 g. Because, like all volatile-oil-containing diuretics, it induces aquaresis by irritating the kidney, the herb should not be used in cases of kidney disease. Further, furocoumarins with photosensitizing properties are present in the oil, so persons using this remedy should avoid prolonged exposure to strong sunlight.

Antiseptic Herbs

Bearberry

The most effective antibacterial herb for urinary tract infections, bearberry is often characterized as a "diuretic," but in fact, its aquaretic properties are minimal. Consisting of the dried leaves of

Arctostaphylos uva-ursi (L.) Spreng, this member of the family Ericaceae is represented in the United States by two principal varieties, *coactylis* and *adenotricha* Fern. & Macbr. For many years it was widely used as a urinary antiseptic as indicated by its status in the official compendia (*USP* and *NF*) from 1820 to 1950.[28] The cessation of its widespread use coincided with the development of sulfa drugs and antibiotics that proved very effective against urinary tract infections.

Bearberry, or uva ursi as it is commonly called, contains a number of constituents including flavonoids, tannins, organic acids, and the like; however, the antiseptic properties of the herb are due to the presence of two phenolic glycosides–arbutin and methylarbutin–which are present in a concentration of about 10 percent.[29] When the plant, or an extract of it, is consumed, arbutin is hydrolyzed in the intestinal tract to yield hydroquinone. Following absorption, this compound is bound as glycuronides and sulfate esters that are excreted in the urine. If the urine is alkaline (over pH 8), the conjugates, especially the sulfate esters, are partially saponified, and the hydroquinone thus freed produces an antibacterial effect.[30]

Obviously, bearberry will be effective only if the urine is maintained at an alkaline pH. This requires consumption of a diet rich in milk, vegetables (especially tomatoes), fruits, fruit juices, potatoes, etc. In addition, consumption of 6 to 8 g. of sodium bicarbonate per day will assure alkalinity. Obviously, it is impractical to maintain an alkaline urine for an extended period of time. This greatly reduces the utility of bearberry as a urinary antiseptic.

The German Commission E recommends bearberry as a treatment for inflammatory conditions of the urinary tract; it is considered to be a bacteriostatic, not an aquaretic.[31] Usual dose is 10 g. (1/3 oz.) daily, corresponding to approximately 400 to 700 mg. of arbutin. Because the leaves are rich in tannin, a suitable beverage is best prepared by soaking the leaves in a quantity of cold water overnight. In this way, much less tannin is dissolved in comparison to a tea prepared with boiling water. Because of the potential toxicity of hydroquinone and the impracticality of maintaining an alkaline urine, bearberry should be utilized for only relatively short periods of time–a few days at most.

Anti-Infective Herbs

Cranberry

One of the most useful herbs for the prevention and treatment of urinary tract infections (UTI), cranberry lacks any antiseptic or antibacterial properties, per se. The sweetened, diluted juice of the American cranberry, *Vaccinium macrocarpon* Ait. (family Ericaceae), also known as the trailing swamp cranberry, is marketed as cranberry juice cocktail. It was reported in 1923 that the urine of test subjects became more acid after eating large amounts of cranberries.[32] Because an acid medium hinders bacterial development, it was postulated that the berries might be useful in preventing or curing UTI, a condition especially prevalent among women. At the time, conventional medical treatments were largely ineffective.

In consequence, many women suffering from this condition began to consume quantities of the cocktail and reported good results. Such word-of-mouth recommendations were supplemented occasionally by articles in regional medical journals. One of the latter reported symptomatic relief from chronic kidney inflammation in female patients who drank 6 ounces (180 ml.) of cranberry juice twice daily. Even though a 1967 study showed that consumption of the commercial cranberry juice cocktail did not appreciably acidify the urine of consumers,[33] UTI sufferers continued to drink it and to report beneficial results.

It is now recognized that the effectiveness of cranberry juice in treating UTI results not from its acidifying properties but as a result of its ability to prevent the microorganisms from adhering to the epithelial cells that line the urinary tract.[34,35] The most common of the UTI-causing bacteria is *Escherichia coli*. It produces two constituents known as adhesins that cause the organism to cling to the epithelial cells where they multiply rapidly. Adhesin activity is inhibited by two different constituents of cranberry juice. One of these is the nearly ubiquitous fructose, but the other is a polymeric compound of unknown identity.[36] Other constituents in cranberry include various carbohydrates and fiber, as well as a number of plant acids, including benzoic, citric, malic, and quinic.[37]

Recommended dosage of cranberry juice cocktail as a UTI preventive is 3 fluidounces or 90 ml. (about one-third of which is pure juice); as a UTI treatment, consumption should be increased into the range of 12 to 32 fluidounces (360-960 ml.) daily. An artificially sweetened product is available if sugar intake is to be limited.

Capsules containing dried cranberry powder are also available; 6 are said to be equivalent to 3 fluidounces (90 ml.) of cocktail. Fresh or frozen cranberries may also be consumed; 1.5 ounces (45 g.) is equivalent to 3 fluidounces (90 ml.) of cocktail. In practice, this is scarcely feasible because of the high acidity and extremely sour taste of the raw berries.

BENIGN PROSTATIC HYPERPLASIA (PROSTATE ENLARGEMENT)

The majority of men who consult urologists do so because of some kind of impairment of the urinary flow. In the group under 45 years of age, this is usually due to prostatitis, that is, an inflammation–frequently an infection–of the prostate gland. In men over 45, the cause is often benign prostatic hyperplasia (BPH) brought about by an abnormal, but nonmalignant, proliferation of cells and tissues of the gland. Eventually, urethral obstruction leads to urinary retention, kidney damage, and infection. In advanced stages, surgical resection is the treatment of choice.

To understand how medications may affect BPH, it is necessary to understand the mechanism that causes the condition. In the prostate, as is the case with many accessory sex organs, testosterone from the blood is converted by the enzyme steroid 5α-reductase to the more potent androgen, dihydrotestosterone (DHT). The DHT binds to a receptor in the cytoplasm and is transferred to the nucleus where it initiates ribonucleic acid (RNA) and deoxyribonucleic acid (DNA) synthesis. This, in turn, results in protein synthesis, cell metabolism, and cell division.[38] In the normal growth process, when sex accessory organs reach a certain size, their further development is no longer influenced by testosterone or DHT. However, $4 \times$ to $6 \times$ the normal amount of DHT is found in the hyperplastic prostate. Apparently, this high concentration of the hormone results in increased growth of the gland in mature males, but the reason for its presence and the manner in which it leads to hyperplasia are poorly understood.[39]

To be most effective in the treatment of BPH, a drug must act to reduce the effects of androgens. It may function by decreasing the amount of hormone produced or available, or it may display a direct antiandrogenic activity and inhibit formation of the DHT-receptor complex in the gland. In addition, anti-inflammatory properties of a drug are significant and certainly may play a secondary role. Estrogens produce androgen ablation by a variety of mechanisms, and their effects of feminization, impotence, and cardiovascular toxicity in the male are highly undesirable. While several plants contain compounds with antiandrogenic and anti-inflammatory properties and are widely used to treat the early stages of BPH in Europe, it must be noted that they cannot be sold for this purpose in the United States. The FDA has banned their sale for two reasons: the agency has not received evidence proving their effectiveness, and their use may delay proper medical treatment.[40] Two of the drugs have, however, received approval by German health authorities.[41]

Saw Palmetto (Sabal)

Saw Palmetto consists of the partially dried, ripe fruit of *Serenoa repens* (Bartr.) Small, a low, scrubby palm of the family Arecaceae that grows from South Carolina to Florida. The name sabal, although frequently applied to this small fan-palm, is now best reserved for the species of usually tall, tree-like palms belonging to the genus *Sabal*. First under the title Sabal, later Serenoa, it was an "official" drug from 1906 to 1950 and was once widely used for a variety of ailments, particularly those of the urogenital type, before falling into near oblivion in this country after World War II.

European scientists, however, continued to study saw palmetto and recognized that, in patients suffering from BPH, an extract of the fruits produced increased urinary flow, reduced residual urine, increased ease in commencing micturition, and decreased frequency of urination.[42] The mechanism of action is antiandrogenic, at least in part. Studies have shown that a liposterolic extract of the berries reduced the uptake by tissue specimens of both testosterone and DHT by more than 40 percent.[43] This mechanism is confirmed by the observation that saw palmetto extract does not induce changes in the level of testosterone, or other hormones, in the plasma itself.[44] Other studies have noted that a plant extract reduces the conversion of less active testosterone to the more active DHT by inhibiting the enzyme steroid 5α-reductase.[45] In addition to their antiandrogenic properties, anti-inflammatory or antiedematous activity has also been demonstrated in the berries. This apparently results from inhibition of the cyclooxygenase and 5-lipoxygenase pathways thereby preventing the biosynthesis of inflammation-producing prostaglandins and leukotrienes. The antiedematous activity in all likelihood is caused by inhibition of the arachidonic acid cascade.

Together, the antiandrogenic and anti-inflammatory effects seem to account for the beneficial role of the herb in treating BPH. Placebo-controlled, double-blind clinical studies carried out on more than 2,000 BPH patients in Germany have confirmed the effectiveness of a saw palmetto extract in such conditions.[46]

Chemical examination of saw palmetto has identified a relatively large number of constituents of the contained volatile and fatty oils including, in the latter, large amounts of β-sitosterol-3-D-glucoside. Various acids, such as anthranilic, caffeic, and chlorogenic, as well as tannin, sugars, and polysaccharides, are also present.[47] Unfortunately, the active antiandrogenic principles remain unidentified, but they are known to reside in the acidic lipophilic fraction of the drupes. A water-soluble polysaccharide was once reported to possess anti-inflammatory properties, but a more recent study found that the polysaccharides, β-sitosterol derivatives, and flavonoids all lacked anti-inflammatory effects when given orally.[48] It thus appears that the principal activity of the fruit resides in the nonpolar constituents.

German health authorities confirm this position by specifying a daily dose of saw palmetto of 1 to 2 g. or 320 mg. of an extract prepared by extracting the drug with a lipophilic solvent such as hexane or 90 percent alcohol. While it is noted that an aqueous extract of the berries possesses antiexudative properties, such action, if present, is minimal in comparison to that of the lipophilic extract. This has important implications for those intending to use the crude drug in the customary form of a tea. Obviously, an aqueous beverage prepared from it would not contain the water-insoluble active constituents, so a preparation of this kind would have little value. For best effect, either the whole drug or an extract prepared with a nonpolar solvent must be used. Once again, the sale of such preparations in the United States is forbidden by the FDA.

Nettle Root

Use of the root of the stinging nettle, *Urtica dioica* L., or the small stinging nettle, *U. urens* L., or hybrids of these members of the family Urticaceae, for treatment of BPH is a relatively recent innovation in phytomedicine. A number of clinical studies support the plant's effectiveness. Chemical analysis of nettle root has resulted in the isolation and identification of a number of low and high molecular weight compounds. The former include various lignans, scopoletin, sitosterol, sitosterol-3-*O*-glucoside, oleanolic acid, and 9-hydroxyl-10-*trans*-12-*cis*-octadecanoic acid. High molecular weight compounds include isolectins and five acid and neutral polysaccharides. The identity of the active principle and, consequently, its mechanism of action remain unknown.[49]

It has been postulated that the herb may have an effect on the amount of free (active) testosterone circulating in the blood, or it may inhibit one of the key enzymes, aromatase, responsible for testosterone synthesis. Another, more recent theory attributes the activity to the presence of a lectin (protein) mixture designated UDA (*Urtica dioica* agglutinin) and several polysaccharides. UDA is unusually stable to acids and heat; consequently, it would retain its activity on oral administration.[50] None of these various postulates regarding nettle root activity is conclusively proven.

German health authorities have concluded that nettle root is an effective treatment for urinary difficulties arising from the early stages of prostate adenoma or BPH.[51] The usual dose is 4 to 6 g. daily. Because the active principles are apparently water soluble, the root may be administered in the form of a tea. Contraindications are unknown and side effects, consisting mostly of gastrointestinal disturbances, are minimal.

The dried leaves of the nettle plant are commonly employed as an aquaretic, and their consumption does result in an increase in the flow of urine.[52] The active principles responsible for this effect have not been identified. **Nettle Leaves** are ordinarily taken in the form of a tea prepared from 3 to 4 teaspoonfuls (about 4 g.) of the botanical and 150 ml. of boiling water. One cup may be drunk 3 to 4 times daily together with additional water. As is the case with other herbal aquaretics, nettle leaf is not effective for hypertension or for edema resulting from cardiac insufficiency.

REFERENCE NOTES

1. Berndt, W.O. and Stitzel, R.E.: "Chapter 20" in *Modern Pharmacology*, C.R. Craig and R.E. Stitzel, eds., Little, Brown, Boston, 1990, pp. 248-270.

2. Schilcher, H. and Emmrich, D.: *Deutsche Apotheker Zeitung* **132**:2549-2555 (1992).

3. Hänsel, R. and Haas, H.: *Therapie mit Phytopharmaka*, Springer-Verlag, Berlin, 1984, p. 206.

4. Schilcher, H.: *Deutsche Apotheker Zeitung* **131**:838-840 (1991).

5. Begg, V.L.: *Herb Quarterly* No. 50: 33-35 (1991)

6. Deam, C.C.: *Flora of Indiana*, State of Indiana Department of Conservation, Division of Forestry, Indianapolis, 1940, pp. 919-928.

7. Schilcher, H., Boesel, R., Effenberger, St., and Segebrecht, S.: *Zeitschrift für Phytotherapie* **10**:77-82 (1989).

8. Wren, R.C.: *Potter's New Cyclopaedia of Botanical Drugs and Preparations*, C.W. Daniel, Saffron Walden, England, 1988, pp. 131-132.

9. Metzner, J., Hirschelmann, R., and Hiller, K.: *Pharmazie* **39**:869-870 (1984).

10. Foetsch, G., Pfeifer, S., Bartoszek, M., Franke, P., and Hiller, K.: *Pharmazie* **44**:555-558 (1989).

11. Chodera, A., et al. (6 other authors): *Acta Poloniae Pharmaceutica* **42**:199-204 (1985).

12. Reznicek, G. et al. (6 other authors): *Planta Medica* **58**:94-98 (1992).

13. Bader, G., Binder, K., Hiller, K., and Ziegler-Böhme, H.: *Pharmazie* **42**:140 (1987).

14. Kraus, J., Schneider, M., and Franz, G.: *Deutsche Apotheker Zeitung* **126**:2045-2049 (1986).

15. Pahlow, M.: *Das grosse Buch der Heilpflanzen*, Gräfe und Unzer, Munich, 1979, p. 147.

16. *Bundesanzeiger* (Cologne, Germany): April 14, 1987; March 6, 1990.

17. *Lawrence Review of Natural Products:* February, 1991.

18. *Bundesanzeiger* (Cologne, Germany): January 5, 1989.

19. Steinegger, E. and Hänsel, R.: *Lehrbuch der Pharmakognosie und Phytopharmazie*, 4th ed., Springer-Verlag, Berlin, 1988, pp. 319-321.

20. Claus, E.P.: *Gathercoal and Wirth Pharmacognosy*, 3rd ed., Lea & Febiger, Philadelphia, 1956, pp. 290-291.

21. Claus, E.P. and Tyler, V.E., Jr.: *Pharmacognosy*, 5th ed., Lea & Febiger, Philadelphia, 1965, pp. 200-201.

22. *Bundesanzeiger* (Cologne, Germany): December 5, 1984.

23. Steinegger E., and Hänsel, R.: *Lehrbuch der Pharmakognosie und Phytopharmazie*, 4th ed., Springer-Verlag, Berlin, 1988, pp. 564-565.

24. Schilcher, H. and Rau, H.: *Urologe B* **28**:274-280 (1988).

25. *Bundesanzeiger* (Cologne, Germany): March 13, 1986.

26. Vollmann, C.: *Zeitschrift für Phytotherapie* **9**:128-132 (1988).

27. *Bundesanzeiger* (Cologne, Germany): June 1, 1990.

28. Claus, E.P. and Tyler, V.E., Jr.: *Pharmacognosy*, 5th ed., Lea & Febiger, Philadelphia, 1965, pp. 152-153.

29. *Lawrence Review of Natural Products:* September, 1987.

30. Steinegger, E. and Hänsel, R.: *Lehrbuch der Pharmakognosie und Phytopharmazie*, 4th ed., Springer-Verlag, Berlin, pp. 696-699.

31. *Bundesanzeiger* (Cologne, Germany): December 5, 1984.

32. Blatherwick, N.R. and Long, M.L.: *Journal of Biological Chemistry* **57**:815-818 (1923).

33. *Lawrence Review of Natural Products:* August, 1987.

34. Sabota, A. E.: *Journal of Urology* **131**:1013-1016 (1984).

35. Soloway, M.S. and Smith, R.A.: *Journal of the American Medical Association* **260**:1465 (1988).

36. Ofek, I., Goldhar, J., Zafriri, D., Lis, H., and Sharon, N.: *New England Journal of Medicine* **324**:1599 (1991).

37. Hughes, B.G. and Lawson, L.D.: *American Journal of Hospital Pharmacy* **46**:1129 (1989).

38. Schwartz, F.L. and Miller, R.J.: "Chapter 67" in *Modern Pharmacology*, 3rd ed., C.R. Craig and R.E. Stitzel, eds., Little, Brown, Boston, 1990, pp. 896-897.

39. Hänsel, R. and Haas, H.: *Therapie mit Phytopharmaka*, Springer-Verlag, Berlin, 1984, p. 201.

40. Anon.: *American Pharmacy* NS **30**:321 (1990).

41. *Bundesanzeiger* (Cologne, Germany): January 5, 1989; February 1, 1990; March 6, 1990.

42. Harnischfeger, G. and Stolze, H.: *Zeitschrift für Phytotherapie* **10**:71-76 (1989).

43. El Sheikh, M.M., Dakkak, M.R., and Saddique, A.: *Acta Obstetrica et Gynecologica Scandinavica* **67**:397-399 (1988).

44. Casarosa, C., Di Coscio, M.C.O., and Fratta, M.: *Clinical Therapeutics* **10**:585-588 (1988).

45. Sultan, C. et al. (6 other authors): *Journal of Steroid Biochemistry* **20**:515-519 (1984).

46. Breu, W., Stadler, F., Hagenlocher, M., and Wagner, H.: *Zeitschrift für Phytotherapie* **13**:107-115 (1992).

47. Hänsel, R. and Haas, H.: *Therapie mit Phytopharmaka*, Springer-Verlag, Berlin, 1984, p. 202.

48. Hiermann, A.: *Archiv der Pharmazie* **322**:111-114 (1989).

49. Goetz, P.: *Zeitschrift für Phytotherapie* **10**:175-178 (1989).

50. Willer, F., Wagner, H., and Schecklies, E.: *Deutsche Apotheker Zeitung* **131**:1217-1221 (1991).

51. *Bundesanzeiger* (Cologne, Germany): January 5, 1989; March 6, 1990.

52. *Bundesanzeiger* (Cologne, Germany): April 23, 1987.

Chapter 6

Respiratory Tract Problems

BRONCHIAL ASTHMA

Bronchial asthma is a condition characterized by difficulty in breathing. It occurs when extrinsic factors (allergens) or intrinsic factors (nonimmunological conditions) cause various mediators, including histamine and the leukotrienes, to be released from mast cells and circulating basophils. This results in relatively rapid contraction of the smooth muscle that surrounds the airways accompanied by a slower secretion of thick, tenacious mucus and edema of the respiratory mucosa. Characterized by wheezing, coughing, shortness of breath, and tightness in the chest, bronchial asthma is reversible. Treatment involves the use of bronchial dilators, the most common of which is theophylline, as well as various adrenergic amines, anticholinergic agents, anti-inflammatory steroids, and the like.[1]

Theophylline occurs with the related xanthine derivatives caffeine and theobromine in several different plant products including coffee, tea, cocoa, and cola. The highest concentration occurs in tea, *Camellia sinensis* (L.) O. Kuntze, but even there it seldom exceeds 0.0004 percent.[2] Consumption of approximately 55 pounds (25 kg.) of tea would be required to equal one 100 mg. tablet of theophylline. When one considers that 6 to 8 times this quantity would be administered daily to relieve an acute attack of bronchial asthma, the impossibility of consuming tea as a source of the necessary theophylline becomes obvious.

Plants containing the solanaceous alkaloids–atropine, hyoscyamine, and scopolamine–reduce bronchospasm by their anticholinergic action. Formerly, the leaves of Jimson weed, *Datura stramonium* L. of the family Solanaceae, were burned and the smoke inhaled to alleviate the condition. Such use has been largely discontinued, not only because of high potential toxicity, but because the alkaloids reduce bronchial secretion and ciliary activity of the bronchial epithelium, thus diminishing the expectorant action needed to clear the respiratory passages.[3]

The only common plant remedy useful for the treatment of bronchial asthma is the following adrenergic herb.

Ephedra

Often referred to by its Chinese name, *ma huang*, ephedra, the green stems of various *Ephedra* species, particularly *E. sinica* Stapf, *E. equisetina* Bunge, and others of the family Ephedraceae, has been used in China for the treatment of bronchial asthma and related conditions for more than 5,000 years. Another species, *E. gerardiana* Wall., has been similarly employed in India. Ephedra was the first Chinese herbal remedy to yield an active constituent, in this case ephedrine, widely used in Western medicine.[4]

Ephedrine was first isolated from the herb by a Japanese chemist, N. Nagai, in 1887. Nearly 40 years elapsed before K. K. Chen and his mentor, C. F. Schmidt, of the Peking Union Medical College began to publish, in 1924, a series of studies on the pharmacological properties of the alkaloid. American physicians were quick to appreciate the adrenergic properties of ephedrine, and it became widely used as a nasal decongestant, a central nervous system stimulant, and a treatment for bronchial asthma.[5] In addition to ephedrine, several other alkaloids, including pseudoephedrine, norephedrine, norpseudoephedrine, etc., are contained in various species of *Ephedra*. These possess physiological properties similar to those of ephedrine.[6]

The approximately 40 different species of *Ephedra* are grouped by Hegnauer into five geographic types based primarily on variations in their alkaloid content.[7] All North American and Central American types appear to be devoid of alkaloids; thus, any activity attributed to these species must derive from compounds other than ephedrine or its derivatives. This is of particular interest in the case of *E. nevadensis* S. Wats., the ingredient in Mormon tea. As an American species of *Ephedra*, it is alkaloid free and of no value in the treatment of bronchial asthma. It should be emphasized that even specialists often find the different species of *Ephedra* difficult to classify.

Chinese ephedra is a relatively potent and useful herb for relieving the constriction associated with asthma. It produces bronchodilation, vasoconstriction, and tends to reduce bronchial edema. In spite of the claims of some advocates,[8] there is no substantial evidence that ephedra is a safe or effective promoter of weight loss in obese persons.

The herb is often administered in the form of a tea prepared by steeping 1 heaping teaspoonful (2 g.) in 1/2 pint (240 ml.) of boiling water for 10 minutes.[9] If prepared from plant material of good quality, this would represent 15 to 30 mg. of ephedrine, which approximates the usual dose of the alkaloid.

Ephedrine is a central nervous system stimulant. It causes an increase in both systolic and diastolic blood pressure as well as heart rate. Large doses may cause nervousness, headache, insomnia, dizziness, palpitations, skin flushing, tingling, and vomiting.[10] These side effects render the indiscriminate use of ephedra highly inadvisable, particularly by persons suffering from heart conditions, hypertension, diabetes, or thyroid disease.

Because of its chemical structure, ephedrine can serve as a precursor for the illegal synthesis of methamphetamine or "speed," a common drug of abuse. Several states have recently passed laws regulating the sale of the alkaloid or products containing it. This concern overlooks the fact that today most ephedrine is produced by a chemical synthesis involving the reductive condensation of L-1-phenyl-1-acetylcarbinol with methylamine. This yields the desired isomer L-ephedrine that is identical in all respects to that contained in ephedra. In view of the difficulties involved in extracting and purifying the relatively small concentrations of ephedrine from the ephedra herb, and the fact that the plant serves only as a minor source of the alkaloid anyway, restricting the availability of the herb, although well intended, seems an excessive measure.[11,12]

COLDS AND FLU

Acute viral infections of the upper respiratory tract produce a mixture of symptoms variously called the "common cold," acute rhinitis, or catarrh. Symptoms of this highly contagious condition include nasal congestion and discharge accompanied by sneezing, irritation, or a "tickling" sensation in the dry or sore throat that gives rise to cough, laryngitis, bronchial congestion, headache, and fever. If the infection is particularly severe and results in significant malaise, including joint and muscle pain and, possibly, gastrointestinal disturbances, the condition is called influenza or "flu." Both conditions are self-limiting (5 to 7 days) but may become complicated by secondary bacterial infections.[13] Further, some symptoms, such as cough, may persist for several weeks.

Treatment of the common cold and flu is largely symptomatic; curative remedies do not exist. In addition to ephedra, which may serve as a useful decongestant, the most effective herbal remedies are those used to treat coughs. These fall into two categories, antitussives (cough suppressants) and expectorants, but the two are closely related, and there is some overlap of herbal products used to treat the condition.

Demulcent Antitussives

Antitussives act either centrally on the medullary cough center of the brain or peripherally at the site of irritation. While some of the best centrally active antitussives, e.g., codeine, are plant products, they are subject to abuse and are not available for self-selection. Consequently, they are not discussed here.

Certain volatile oils obtained from herbs are incorporated into a sugar base and marketed in the form of lozenges to suppress coughs. Some of the more popular oils used for this purpose include anise, eucalyptus, fennel, peppermint, and thyme. Cough drops flavored with these oils apparently function by stimulating the formation and secretion of saliva, which produces more frequent swallowing and thereby tends to suppress the cough reflex.[14] However, the real therapeutic utility of volatile-oil-containing herbs in treating conditions associated with colds and flu is their expectorant action. The effective herbal expectorants will be considered following the antitussives.

The antitussive effect of many herbs results from the content of mucilage, which exerts a demulcent or protective action. Mucilages are hydrophilic colloids that, in the presence of water, tend to form viscous solutions–or tacky gels. When consumed, usually in the form of a tea, they form a protective layer over the mucous membrane of the pharynx, larynx, and trachea, thereby preventing mechanical irritation of the receptors there and preventing the cough reflex. Since the mucilage is not absorbed and its action is essentially a mechanical one, it does not produce untoward side effects. However, some mucilage-containing herbs possess additional constituents that are toxic. This is the case with one of the long-used herbal antitussives, **Coltsfoot**, the leaves of *Tussilago farfara* L. of the family Asteraceae. Although coltsfoot has useful cough-protective properties, its use cannot be recommended because it also contains toxic pyrrolizidine alkaloids (PAs).

The following mucilage-containing antitussive herbs may be employed more or less interchangeably and are listed in alphabetical order.

Iceland Moss

Not a higher plant, but a lichen–that is, an alga and a fungus growing in symbiotic association–Iceland moss is obtained from *Cetraria islandica* (L.) Ach. of the family Parmeliaceae. Commercial supplies of this foliaceous lichen are obtained primarily from Scandinavia and central Europe. It contains about 50 percent of a mixture of mucilaginous polysaccharides, principally lichenin and isolichenin.[15] Iceland moss is consumed in the form of a decoction prepared from 1 to 2 heaping teaspoonfuls (1.5-3 g.) of herb and 150 ml. of water. Drink 1 cup 3 times a day.[16] Total daily dose is 4 to 6 g. of plant material. The German Commission E has found Iceland moss effective for the treatment of irritations of the mouth and throat and associated dry cough.[17]

A recent study by Finnish scientists warns against utilizing Iceland moss in large quantities over an extended period of time. It has long been used as an emergency food in that country, but in recent years the lead content of the lichen has increased to the point (30 mg. per kg. dry weight) where this practice can no longer be considered safe.[18] While the relatively small amounts used occasionally for the treatment of cough probably pose negligible risk, it is nevertheless a concern about which consumers should be aware.

Marshmallow Root

This herb consists of the dried root, deprived of the brown outer corky layer, of *Althaea officinalis* L. (family Malvaceae). It contains 5 to 10 percent of mucilage and is consumed in the form of a tea, 1 to 2 teaspoonfuls (5-10 g.) in 150 ml. of water (daily dose–6 g.), for its antitussive effect.[14] In Europe, the leaves of this plant, as well as the leaves and flowers of the common mallow, *Malva sylvestris* L., and related species and subspecies, are all employed similarly. Commission E has declared them all to be effective demulcents.[17]

Mullein Flowers

The flowers of several species of mullein, *Verbascum thapsus* L., *V. densiflorum* Bertol., and *V. phlomoides* L. (family Scrophulariaceae), all contain about 3 percent of a mucilage useful in the treatment of throat irritations and cough. The flowers (3-4 teaspoonfuls or 1.5-2 g.) are used to prepare 150 ml. of tea, which may be drunk several times daily.[14] Approved by Commission E for the treatment of respiratory catarrh, the herb also has some expectorant activity.[19]

Plantain Leaves

Fresh or dried leaves of the English plantain, *Plantago lanceolata* L. (family Plantaginaceae), have a worldwide reputation as a soothing cough suppressant.[20] This action is attributed primarily to the approximately 6 percent of mucilage found in the plant material; tannins and bitter principles may contribute as well. The herb is also employed for inflammatory conditions of the oral cavity as well as to treat various skin inflammations.

Plantain's effectiveness in these latter conditions is due in part to its mucilage content, but in addition, two iridoid glycosides–aucubin and catapol–almost certainly play a role, at least under certain conditions. When the sap is expressed from the fresh leaves, the glycosides are hydrolyzed, and the residual aglycones exert a strong antibacterial effect. This accounts for the folkloric use of the fresh crushed leaves as an anti-inflammatory and wound-healing agent.

Of course, the antibacterial products are not present in the infusions customarily used to relieve coughs because boiling water inactivates the hydrolytic enzyme.[21] German Commission E has found plantain safe and effective as a soothing demulcent, astringent, and antibacterial.[22] It is customarily administered as a tea prepared from 3 to 4 teaspoonfuls (2-3 g.) of the herb and 150 ml. of boiling water.

Slippery Elm

Indians and early settlers of North America valued the inner bark of the slippery elm, *Ulmus rubra* Muhl. (family Ulmaceae), as a poultice and soothing drink. The bark of this large tree, native to the eastern and central United States, contains large quantities of a viscid mucilage that acts as an effective demulcent and antitussive.[23] While the herb may be consumed in the form of a tea, a number of throat lozenges containing it are commercially available. These are the preferred dosage form for the treatment of cough and minor throat irritations because they provide a sustained release of the mucilage to the pharynx.

This native American herb has not seen widespread usage elsewhere, so European authorities have not commented on its safety and efficacy. Some measure of its utility may be gathered from the fact that it was listed in the official compendia (*USP* and *NF*) from 1820 to 1960.[24] The FDA has declared it to be a safe and effective oral demulcent.

Expectorants

Prolonged irritation of the bronchioles results in an increase in the mucoprotein and acidic mucopolysaccharide content of their secretions and a concomitant increase in the viscosity of the mucus and other fluids. This and several related factors reduce the ability of ciliary movement and coughing to move the thickened secretions toward the pharynx. Symptomatic therapy with expectorants has the objective of reducing the viscosity of these secretions so that the loosened material may be eliminated from the system, eventually by expectoration.

The action of the so-called nauseant-expectorant herbs that contain alkaloids results primarily from their action on the gastric mucosa. This provokes a reflex stimulation of the vomiting center in the brain via the vagus nerve, which leads to an increase in secretion of the bronchial glands. Volatile-oil type expectorant herbs, on the other hand, exert a direct stimulatory effect on the bronchial glands by means of local irritation. Saponin-containing expectorant herbs function by reducing the surface tension of the secretions, facilitating their separation from the mucous membranes.[25] Of course, some expectorant herbs combine two or more of these effects. For example, the saponin-containing senega root also possesses nauseant-expectorant properties.

Use of expectorants is based primarily on tradition. Subjectively, they appear to be effective for the treatment of irritative, nonproductive coughs associated with a small amount of secretion. Substantial proof of their therapeutic utility is lacking. Nevertheless, they form a significant group of herbal remedies, and some appear to be of value. In the following discussion, they are classified on the basis of their mode of action: (1) nauseant-expectorants, (2) local irritants, and (3) surface-tension modifiers. The classification is imprecise because the function of many of the herbs is incompletely understood, and some play a multiplicity of roles.

Nauseant-Expectorants

The two most effective nauseant-expectorant herbs cannot be used extemporaneously because of their potential toxicity and the need to administer their active constituents in precise doses.

Ipecac

The first of these is Ipecac. This consists of the rhizome and roots of *Cephaelis ipecacuanha* (Brot.) A. Rich. or *C. acuminata* Karst. of the family Rubiaceae.[26] Ipecac Syrup (*USP*) is widely used as an emetic in the treatment of certain poisonings, but it is prepared from Powdered Ipecac (*USP*), which is standardized to contain from 1.9 to 2.1 percent of the active ether-soluble ipecac alkaloids, primarily emetine, caphaeline, and psychotrine. A number of commercial expectorant mixtures also contain precise amounts of standardized ipecac, and these are the preferred dosage form of this useful expectorant. Follow the directions on the label.

Lobelia

A second effective herbal nauseant-expectorant, which cannot be used safely because standardized preparations do not exist, is lobelia. Commonly called Indian tobacco, it consists of the leaves and tops of *Lobelia inflata* L., family Campanulaceae. This native American plant was at one time widely used in this country by so-called lobelia doctors who practiced a system of medicine developed by Samuel Thomson in the early nineteenth century. Lobelia, as a result of its contained alkaloids, principally lobeline, is an effective nauseant-expectorant, but the ratio of risk to benefit is very high. Its use as a crude herbal product is not recommended.[27]

Local Irritants

Two effective volatile-oil-containing expectorant herbs, **Anise** and **Fennel**, have been previously discussed (see Chapter 4, "Digestive System Problems," for details).

Horehound

Possibly the most effective and pleasant-tasting plant drug in this category is horehound. Consisting of the leaves and flowering tops of *Marrubium vulgare* L. (family Lamiaceae), horehound has been used as a cough remedy for some 400 years. It also has choleretic properties, so it serves to facilitate digestion as well. The activity of the herb is attributed not only to its content (0.06 percent) of volatile oil, but especially to a bitter diterpenoid lactone, marrubiin (or its possible precursor in the plant, premarrubiin). This compound exerts a direct stimulatory effect on the secretions of the bronchial mucosa.[28]

In 1989, the FDA banned horehound from over-the-counter cough remedies because it had not received sufficient evidence supporting its efficacy. It is still on the GRAS list, however, and in 1990, the German Commission E approved horehound for the treatment of bronchial catarrh as well as dyspepsia and loss of appetite.[19]

Horehound may be consumed as a tea prepared from 2 heaping teaspoonfuls (2 g.) of the cut herb steeped in 240 ml. of boiling water. Three to 5 cups (0.75-1 liter) may be consumed daily; untoward side effects have not been reported.[29] The herb is also available in the form of hard horehound candy that is widely used as a cough lozenge.

Thyme

This is another useful irritant-expectorant herb. The leaves and tops of two different species of *Thymus* (family Lamiaceae) are now used more or less interchangeably. These are *T. vulgaris* L. (common or garden thyme) and *T. zygis* L. (Spanish thyme). However, it must be noted that common thyme contains a greater quantity of volatile oil (0.4-3.4 percent) than Spanish thyme (0.7-1.38 percent), so equivalent weights are not equivalent therapeutically. The principal constituents of the oil are various phenols, especially thymol (30.7-70.9 percent) and carvacrol (2.5-14.6 percent). Flavonoids are also present in thyme.[30]

The volatile oil has not only expectorant and antiseptic properties but functions to relieve bronchospasm as well.[31] This spasmolytic effect is enhanced by the flavonoids in the plant.[32] Commission E has found thyme to be effective for the treatment of the symptoms of bronchitis, pertussis, and catarrh.[33] It is normally consumed as a tea prepared from 1 to 2 g. (1 teaspoonful) of the herb per cup (240 ml.) of water, and this quantity of the moderately warm tea is drunk up to 3 times daily. It may be sweetened with honey, which also acts as a demulcent, thereby increasing the tea's effectiveness.

Eucalyptus Leaves

Although relatively little-used in comparison to the volatile oil obtained from them, the leaves of *Eucalyptus globulus* Labill. (family Myrtaceae) and related species do possess a useful expectorant activity. To be effective medicinally, the leaf oil must contain 70 to 85 percent cineole (eucalyptol). This is an important criterion because, while there are many species and chemical races of the genus that yield 3 to 6 percent volatile oil, some of them do not contain sufficient cineole to provide the necessary expectorant and antiseptic activity.[34]

A tea prepared from 1/2 teaspoonful (2-3 g.) of eucalyptus leaves in about 150 ml. of hot water, drunk freshly prepared 3 times daily, serves as a useful cough remedy. The volatile oil, which has official status in the *NF*, is commonly incorporated in a variety of nasal inhalers and sprays, balms and ointments (rubs) for external application, and mouthwashes.

Surface-Tension Modifiers

Of the small number of effective saponin-containing expectorant herbs, two are not commonly used in the United States. The leaves of **Ivy**, *Hedera helix* L. (family Araliaceae), cannot be employed as a tea, and the concentrated extracts available in Europe are not articles of commerce in this country. The flowers and root of **Primula**, *Primula veris* L. or *P. elatior* (L.) Hill of the family Primulaceae, are very popular in Europe but not readily available here.[35]

Licorice (Glycyrrhiza), which is widely used in this country, has very useful expectorant or antitussive properties. It has already been discussed as a treatment for stomach ulcers. Although licorice does contain saponins, its mode of action in the treatment of upper respiratory congestion and coughs requires considerable clarification.[35]

Senega Snakeroot

The only significant herb remaining in this category is senega snakeroot. Variously known as senega or seneca root, this herb consists of the dried root of *Polygala senega* L. (family Polygalaceae). The plant is native to the eastern woodlands of North America. It was used by the Seneca Indians to treat rattlesnake bite; hence, the name.

Senega snakeroot contains 5 to 10 percent of a mixture of triterpenoid saponins, which are the active expectorant principles. The major components of the mixture are senegin, also known as poly-galin, and polygalic acid. While these probably function directly to reduce the viscosity of thickened bronchial secretions, their primary mechanism of action appears to be that of a nauseant-expectorant. Irritation of the gastric mucosa leads, by reflex stimulation, to an increase in bronchial mucous gland secretion.[36]

The herb is administered in the form of a decoction prepared from 0.5 g. (about 1/5 teaspoonful) and 1 cup (240 ml.) of water. Total daily dose should not exceed 3 g. because of the tendency of large doses to upset the stomach and to produce nausea and diarrhea. Commission E has approved senega snakeroot as an expectorant for the treatment of upper respiratory catarrh.[37] The drug was official in the *NF* until 1960.

SORE THROAT

Often, but not necessarily, associated with colds and flu, sore throat may be a symptom of many illnesses. These range from acute simple (catarrhal) pharyngitis, usually caused by bacterial or viral infections of the upper respiratory tract, to severe streptococcal infections. It also accompanies certain acute specific infections, such as measles and whooping cough. The kind of dry sore throat that attends colds and flu is usually self-limiting; treatment is symptomatic with emphasis on increasing the patient's comfort. Gargling with warm infusions or decoctions of various herbs is often recommended. The antiseptic and astringent botanicals commonly used as palliatives are essentially the same as those employed for lesions and infections of the oral mucosa. These are discussed together in Chapter 11.

REFERENCE NOTES

1. McPhillips, J.J.: "Chapter 45" in *Modern Pharmacology*, 3rd ed., C. R. Craig and R.E. Stitzel, eds., Little, Brown, Boston, 1990, pp. 601-602.

2. List, P.H. and Hörhammer, L., eds.: *Hagers Handbuch der Pharmazeutisch-en Praxis*, 4th ed., vol. 3, Springer-Verlag, Berlin, 1973, p. 639.

3. Haas, H.: *Arzneipflanzenkunde*, B.I. Wissenschaftsverlag, Mannheim, 1991, p. 64.

4. Osol, A. and Farrar, G.E., Jr.: *The Dispensatory of the United States of America*, 24th ed., J.B. Lippincott, Philadelphia, 1947, pp. 403-407.

5. Kreig, M.B.: *Green Medicine*, Rand McNally, Chicago, 1964, pp. 415-416.

6. Steinegger, E. and Hänsel, R.: *Lehrbuch der Pharmakognosie und Phytopharmazie*, Springer-Verlag, Berlin, 1988, pp. 450-453.

7. Hegnauer, R.: *Chemotaxonomie der Pfanzen*, vol. 1, Birkhäuser Verlag, Basel, 1962, pp. 460-462.

8. Weiner, M.: *Health Foods Business* 37(6):18-20 (1991).

9. Pahlow, M.: *Das grosse Buch der Heilpflanzen*, Gräfe und Unzer, Munich, 1985, pp. 387-388.

10. *Lawrence Review of Natural Products:* June, 1989.

11. Anon.: *Health Foods Business* 37(6):8 (1991)

12. Anon.: *Health Foods Business* 37(8):12 (1991).

13 Bryant, B.G. and Lombardi, T.P.: "Chapter 8" in *Handbook of Nonprescription Drugs*, 9th ed., American Pharmaceutical Association, Washington, D.C., 1990, pp. 136-141.

14. Hänsel, R.: *Phytopharmaka*, 2nd ed., Springer-Verlag, Berlin, 1991, pp. 99-104.

15. Wren, R.C.: *Potter's New Cyclopaedia of Botanical Drugs and Preparations*, rev. ed., C.W. Daniel, Saffron Walden, England, 1988, p 152

16 Pahlow, M.: *Das grosse Buch der Heilpflanzen*, Gräfe and Unzer, Munich, 1985, p. 180.

17. *Bundesanzeiger* (Cologne, Germany): January 5, 1989.

18. Airaksinen, M.M., Peura, P., and Ontere, S.: *Archives of Toxicology* Suppl. 9:406-409 (1986)

19. *Bundesanzeiger* (Cologne, Germany): February 1, 1990.

20. Pahlow, M.: *Heilpflanzen in der Apotheke*, Deutscher Apotheker Verlag, Stuttgart, 1985, pp. 16-17.

21. Wichtl, M.: *Deutsche Apotheker Zeitung* (Supplement *Videopharm*) 125(38):20 (1985).

22. *Bundesanzeiger* (Cologne, Germany): November 30, 1985.

23. *Lawrence Review of Natural Products:* March, 1991.

24. Claus, E.P. and Tyler, V.E., Jr.: *Pharmacognosy*, 5th ed., Lea & Febiger, Philadelphia, 1965, p. 85.

25. Haas, H.: *Arzneipflanzenkunde*, B.I. Wissenschaftsverlag, Mannheim, 1991, pp. 65-72.

26. Tyler, V.E., Brady, L.R., Robbers, J.E.: *Pharmacognosy*, 9th ed., Lea & Febiger, Philadelphia, 1988, pp. 209-212.

27. Tyler, V.E.: *The Honest Herbal*, 3rd ed., Pharmaceutical Products Press, New York, 1993, pp. 205-206.

28. Ibid., pp. 127-128.

29. Pahlow, M.: *Heilpflanzen in der Apotheke*, Deutscher Apotheker Verlag, Stuttgart, 1985, p. 55.

30. List, P.H. and Horhämmer, L., eds.: *Hager's Handbuch der Pharmazeutischen, Praxis*, Springer-Verlag, Berlin, vol. 6C, pp. 161-173.

31. Reiter, M. and Brandt, W.: *Arzneimittelforschung* 35(I):408-414 (1985).

32. Van den Broucke, C.O. and Lemli, J.A.: *Pharmaceutisch Weekblad, Scientific Edition* 5:9-14 (1983).

33. *Bundesanzeiger* (Cologne, Germany): December 5, 1984; March 6, 1990.

34. Tyler, V.E., Brady, L.R., and Robbers, J.E.: *Pharmacognosy*, 9th ed., Lea & Febiger, Philadelphia, 1988, pp. 133-135.

35. Hänsel, R.: *Phytopharmaka*, 2nd ed., Springer-Verlag, Berlin, 1991, pp. 105-120.

36. Briggs, C.J.: *Canadian Pharmaceutical Journal* 121:199-201 (1988).

37. *Bundesanzeiger* (Cologne, Germany): March 13, 1986; March 6, 1990.

Chapter 7

Cardiovascular System Problems

CONGESTIVE HEART FAILURE (CHF)

This is a relatively common clinical disorder in which the heart fails to provide an adequate blood flow to the peripheral tissues of the body. It is a serious condition. Some one-half million Americans suffer from CHF; the five-year survival rate of such patients is less than 50 percent. CHF symptoms are associated with one or more of five key pathophysiologic features. These include blood pressure overload, volume overload, loss of heart muscle, decreased contractility, and disturbances in filling of the heart.[1] When such conditions result in reduced cardiac output, several compensatory mechanisms are activated that may sustain performance for a limited period, but without appropriate drug intervention, cardiac efficiency soon declines. The resulting symptoms include both ankle and pulmonary edema as well as ascites.

Herbs Containing Potent Cardioactive Glycosides

During this century, the drugs utilized most frequently by physicians for the treatment of CHF have been obtained from **Digitalis**, the dried leaves of *Digitalis purpurea* L. and **Digitalis Lanata**, the dried leaves of *D. lanata* Erh. These members of the plant family Scrophulariaceae yield several potent cardiac glycosides, especially digitoxin, which is derived from both, and digoxin, which is prepared only from *D. lanata*. These two glycosides now account for all of the digitalis prescriptions normally dispensed in the United States. However, a standardized *D. purpurea* leaf preparation, Powdered Digitalis, is official in the *USP* and is still employed, along with similar products, in other countries.

Numerous other plants contain cardioactive glycosides with steroidal structures and physiological functions similar to those of digitalis. Some of these have been used from time to time in the treatment of CHF, but none presents any special advantage over digitalis, so only the names and botanical origins of some of the more common ones are listed here:

Adonis–*Adonis vernalis* L., family Ranunculaceae;

Apocynum or **Black Indian Hemp**–*Apocynum cannabinum* L. or *A. androsaemifolium* L., family Ranunculaceae;

Black Hellebore–*Helleborus niger* L., family Ranunculaceae;

Cactus Grandiflorus–*Selenicereus grandiflorus* (L.) Britt. & Rose, family Cactaceae;

Convallaria or **Lily-of-the-Valley**–*Convallaria majalis* L., family Convallariaceae;

Oleander–*Nerium oleander* L., family Apocynaceae;

Squill–*Urginea maritima* (L.) Bak., family Liliaceae; and

Strophanthus–*Strophanthus kombé* Oliv. or *S. hispidus* DC., family Apocynaceae.[3]

CHF is a serious disturbance of multiple origins; it requires prompt, accurate diagnosis and careful treatment. The cardiac glycosides are extremely potent drugs, the dosage of which must be carefully adjusted to the needs of the individual patient. In the case of phytomedicines containing them, this is possible only with the standardized Powdered Digitalis, a product not readily available in the United States. Because nonprofessional diagnosis and treatment of congestive heart failure are not in the best interest of the patient, the names and sources of the herbal products employed to treat it are listed here only for the record, and no further details concerning their use are provided.

ANGINA

Adequate coronary blood flow is vital for normal cardiac function, and the inability of that flow to adjust to myocardial oxygen demands results in the painful condition known as angina or angina pectoris. An inadequate blood flow may result either from coronary artery spasm (primary angina), or from the inability of diseased, partially blocked coronary arteries to meet an increased demand for oxygen (secondary angina), or from a combination of both factors.

Regardless of type, angina is now routinely treated with drugs from three different groups that are effective in reducing both its severity and frequency. Nitrates are especially helpful in providing rapid relief from acute attacks; β-adrenergic receptor antagonists (β-blockers) and slow calcium channel blockers are rational treatments for both vasospastic and effort-induced angina, but the latter drugs are especially useful in the prophylaxis of coronary vasospasm.[4]

The plant kingdom does not yield any drugs that are as effective for the treatment of angina as the nitrates, β-blockers, and calcium channel blockers. Therefore, the use of any herbal remedies in the treatment of this condition is restricted to prevention or, possibly, to follow-up treatment.[5]

Hawthorn

One such herb, widely used in Europe, and enthusiastically recommended by some authorities there, is hawthorn. This herb consists of the leaves with flowers and/or fruits of *Crataegus laevigata* (Poir.) DC. or *C. monogyna* Jacq. of the family Rosaceae. The principal activity of these plant materials is attributed to their content of oligomeric procyanidins with additional effects provided by various flavonoids, including quercetin, hy-peroside, vitexin, and vitexin rhamnoside. Other constituents include catechin and epicatechin.[6]

Accurate evaluation of the utility of hawthorn is difficult because most of the pharmacological and clinical studies of it have been conducted utilizing standardized extracts prepared by methods the details of which are proprietary information.[2] Still, it appears that the herb causes a direct dilation of the smooth muscles of the coronary vessels, thereby lowering their resistance and increasing blood flow. The tendency toward angina is thus reduced. It is, however, not useful for acute attacks because its effects develop quite slowly following continued consumption. Hawthorn is also characterized as having positive inotropic effects; further, it accelerates the heart rate and increases nerve conductivity and heart muscle irritability.[7]

Although Commission E has approved the use of hawthorn for a number of mild cardiac conditions, the minimal daily dosage is

established either on the basis of flavone (5 mg.), total flavonoids
(10 mg.), or oligomeric procyanidins calculated as epicatechin (5
mg.). Since standardized extracts providing these dosage levels are
not available in the United States, and since the wisdom of self-
treating any abnormal heart condition is highly questionable, the
use of such a remedy–even one as devoid of side effects as this
one–cannot be recommended.

ARTERIOSCLEROSIS

Hyperlipoproteinemia, commonly known simply as "high cholesterol" and referring to the concentration of protein-bound cholesterol and triglycerides in the blood plasma, is one of the risk
factors predisposing persons to arteriosclerosis. Three other factors
are diabetes mellitus, smoking, and hypertension.[8] Arteriosclerosis
tends to be a generalized condition involving all major arteries to
some degree with critical involvement of only a few. It is characterized by a gradual narrowing and ultimate occlusion of the affected
vessels, often accompanied by weakening of the arterial walls. The
type of arteriosclerosis characterized by discrete deposits of fatty
substances (atheromatous plaques) in the arteries and by fibrosis
and calcification of their inner layer is called atherosclerosis. Ath-
erosclerotic involvement of the coronary arteries is known as coronary artery disease. It may lead eventually to a sufficient obstruction of the vessels to produce ischemic heart disease accompanied
by angina pectoris and, subsequently, myocardial infarction (heart
attack).

It is interesting that the only herb shown to reduce cholesterol
levels also enhances blood fibrinolytic activity and inhibits platelet
aggregation. There is some evidence to support the claim that it may
even lower blood pressure. All of these actions would be beneficial
in the prevention and treatment of arteriosclerosis and its consequences. The herb is discussed below.

Garlic

Consisting of the bulb of *Allium sativum* L., family Liliaceae,
garlic has been consumed both as a food and a medicine since the

time of the Egyptian pharaohs and the earliest Chinese dynasties. It has been extensively investigated both scientifically and clinically. Well over 1,000 papers on garlic and related alliums have been published in the last 20 years.[9]

The intact cells of garlic contain an odorless, sulfur-containing amino acid derivative known as alliin [(+)-S-allyl-L-cysteine sulfoxide]. When the cells are crushed, it comes into contact with the enzyme alliinase located in neighboring cells and is converted to allicin (diallyl thiosulfinate). Allicin is a potent antibiotic, but it is also highly odoriferous and unstable, yielding, depending on the conditions (steam distillation, oil maceration, etc.), a number of other strong-smelling sulfur compounds, such as: various diallyl sulfides, including mono-, di-, tri-, tetra-, penta-, and hexa-; various methyl allyl sulfides, including mono-, di-, tri-, tetra-, penta-, and hexa-; various dimethyl sulfides, including mono-, di-, tri-, tetra-, penta-, and hexa-; 2-vinyl-4H-1,3-dithiin, 3 vinyl-4H 1,2-dithiin, E-ajoene, and Z-ajoene. The ajoenes are apparently responsible for much of the antithrombotic properties of garlic. Aside from them and the known antibiotic activity of allicin, connections between specific chemical compounds yielded by garlic and its therapeutic properties are not necessarily well established. However, an extensive list of tentative attributions has appeared.[10] Allicin is described there as possessing antiplatelet, antibiotic, and antihyperlipidemic activity. In consequence, most authorities now agree that the best measure of the total activity of garlic is its ability to produce allicin which, in turn, results in the formation of other active principles. This ability is referred to as the allicin yield of the garlic preparation.

Dutch investigators have evaluated the methodologies and results of 18 controlled trials dealing with the beneficial effects of garlic on presumed cardiovascular risk indicators in humans, specifically, reduction of cholesterol, increased fibrinolytic activity, and inhibition of platelet aggregation. They concluded that for fresh garlic the claims are valid but only at relatively high dosage levels. Most studies involved ingestion of 0.25 to 1 g. of fresh garlic per kilogram of body weight per day. This is equivalent to a range of approximately 5 to 20 average-sized (4 g.) cloves of garlic daily for a 175-pound person. Results with commercial garlic preparations were equivocal, as might be expected from dosage forms so diverse in their mode of preparation and constituents. Interestingly, fresh onions also yielded contradictory results, except for an increased fibrinolytic activity that was consistently observed.[10]

In spite of their acceptance of the positive results, these investigators were highly critical of the methodology of most of the 18 studies. However, under the strict guidelines applied by them, it would not be possible to justify the validity of consuming any drug that lowered cholesterol, inhibited platelet aggregation, or increased fibrinolytic activity as a means of ameliorating arteriosclerosis and coronary artery disease. The important conclusion is that fresh garlic in large amounts does produce all of those effects believed by many authorities to be useful preventive measures.

Some recent investigations seem to indicate that much smaller doses of garlic than the 5 or more cloves daily suggested in the Dutch evaluation are nevertheless effective in the treatment of hyperlipidemia. A 16-week study involving 261 patients with total cholesterol and/or triglyceride values exceeding 200 mg. per dl. showed that daily administration of 800 mg. of garlic powder (standardized to 1.3 percent allicin content) reduced cholesterol values by an average of 12 percent and triglyceride values, 17 percent.[11] Assuming that fresh garlic yields, on the average, 0.37 percent allicin, the 10.4 mg. contained in the 800 mg. of garlic powder ingested daily is equivalent to only 2.8 g. of fresh garlic–less than one average-sized clove.

Discussing the effectiveness of commercial garlic preparations is like talking about the *cause* of cancer. They are so variable in their mode of preparation and resulting constituents that each would have to be addressed individually. However, there are a few basic principles. Even carefully dried garlic contains no allicin, the apparent direct precursor of the active constituents and the carrier of the antibiotic activity. It does contain alliin and the enzyme alliinase, which is capable of converting alliin to allicin. But alliinase is inactivated by acids, so no conversion to allicin occurs in the stomach. Fresh garlic quickly releases allicin in the mouth during the chewing process, not in the stomach.[12]

Dried garlic preparations are most effective if the tablets or capsules are enteric coated so that they pass through the stomach and release their contents in the alkaline medium of the small intestine where enzymatic conversion to allicin can readily occur. Once released, the allicin reacts rapidly with the amino acid cysteine derived from proteinaceous food consumed with the garlic. The *S*-allylmercaptocysteine thus formed effectively binds the odoriferous allicin, preventing it from reaching the bloodstream as such. When administered in this way, carefully dried garlic powder is probably relatively effective but produces little garlicky taste or odor.[13]

The activity of other garlic preparations is questionable, particularly those with an oil base. Allicin is unstable in oil, so much of the sulfide content and, consequently, much of the activity of such garlic preparations is lost. A Japanese preparation, consisting of minced garlic aged in aqueous alcohol for 18 to 20 months, contained no detectable levels of allicin or its degradation products. In water, allicin is slowly converted to a number of volatile polysulfides that are also present in the steam-distilled oil. That oil, although high in total sulfides, contains neither allicin nor ajoene. It is obvious that the therapeutic value of various commercial garlic preparations, which appears to be directly related to the product's allicin yield, is highly dependent on the method of preparation, details of which are ordinarily unavailable.[14]

A 1992 study in Germany of 18 of the approximately 70 garlic preparations commercially available in that country revealed that only five produced an allicin yield equivalent to 4 g. of fresh garlic. That is the amount of fresh garlic, or its equivalent, established by German health authorities as the average daily dose required for therapeutic utility. The other 13 preparations were so lacking in active principles as to be designated "expensive placebos." These findings are particularly significant in view of the fact that, in 1990, the garlic preparation market in the German Federal Republic amounted to approximately $160 million. It is estimated that 12 percent of all German citizens over the age of 14 now consume garlic in prepared dosage forms.[15]

Consumption of moderate amounts of garlic does not pose a health risk for normal persons. The larger quantities thought by some to be required for therapeutic purposes (in excess of 5 cloves daily) can result in heartburn, flatulence, and related gastrointestinal problems. Allergies have also been reported, and those taking other anticoagulant drugs should consume garlic with caution.

In addition to its effectiveness in reducing some of the risk factors associated with arteriosclerosis and, specifically, coronary artery disease, garlic may have utility in the treatment of digestive ailments, bacterial and fungal infections, hypertension, and even cancer.[16] Additional studies on the constituents and therapeutic utility of this interesting plant are certainly warranted. At present, its use is approved by the German Commission E to support dietetic measures for the treatment of hyperlipoproteinemia and to prevent age-related changes in the blood vessels (arteriosclerosis).[17]

PERIPHERAL VASCULAR DISEASE

Peripheral vascular disease (PVD) is a general term that includes any disease of the blood vessels outside the heart and thoracic aorta; it also covers disease of the lymph vessels. Three specific types are of special concern because they may respond to treatment with herbal remedies. These are: (1) cerebrovascular disease, (2) other peripheral arterial circulatory disturbances, and (3) venous disorders.[18]

Cerebrovascular Disease

Cerebrovascular disease results from abnormalities of the vessels, such as atherosclerosis or arteritis, or from abnormalities of blood flow or of the blood itself. Changes in blood flow result not only from disease of the vessels but also from thrombotic or embolic processes. Such changes in the brain may produce a reduction in the blood flow, that is, in a condition designated ischemia. The degree of ischemia and its duration vary greatly.[19] Depending on its severity, location, and duration, it may result in numerous unpleasant symptoms frequently experienced by elderly persons, including dizziness, depression, tinnitus, short-term memory loss, and even dementia.

Ginkgo

An herb that has shown considerable promise in alleviating many of these symptoms is Ginkgo. A concentrated extract (GBE) of the leaves of *Ginkgo biloba* L., family Ginkgoaceae, is currently enjoying enormous popularity in Europe as a treatment for peripheral vascular disease, particularly cerebral circulatory disturbances and certain other peripheral arterial circulatory disorders. Although the ginkgo tree is a very old one, having survived unchanged in China for some 200 million years, the herbal remedy prepared from its leaves is quite new, having been developed in the last 20 years. The leaves themselves cannot be used as an extemporaneous herbal remedy, for example, in the form of a tea, because they would provide an insufficient quantity of the active principles. As noted, GBE is widely used; 5.24 million prescriptions for it were written in Germany alone in 1988. GBE is also available there as an over-the-counter drug.[20]

To supply the market with adequate supplies of leaves, plantations of ginkgo trees, severely pruned to shrub height to allow mechanical picking, have been established. The plantation in Sumter, South Carolina, comprises 10 million ginkgos on 1,000 acres.[21] The leaves are picked green, dried, and shipped to Europe for processing. There, an acetone-water extract is prepared, dried, and adjusted to a potency of 24 percent flavone glycosides and 6 percent terpenes.

Although complete analyses of GBE have not been conducted, the extract does contain a number of flavonol and flavone glycosides, principally glycosides of quercetin and kaempferol; rutin is also present. The extract also contains 3 percent or more of a group of unique, closely related, bitter, 20-carbon diterpene lactone derivatives known as ginkgolides A, B, C, and M. In addition, about 3 percent of a similar 15-carbon sesquiterpene designated bilobalide is also present together with 6-hydroxykynurenic acid, shikimic acid, protocatechuic acid, vanillic acid, and *p*-hydroxybenzoic acid.[22]

The therapeutic effects of GBE are attributed to a mixture of these constituents, not to a single chemical entity. Flavones of the rutin type reduce capillary fragility and increase the threshold of blood loss from the capillary vessels. This tends to prevent ultrastructural (ischemic) brain damage. They also function as free-radical scavengers, tending to inhibit the lipid peroxidation of cell membranes by inactivating free oxygen radicals.

Ginkgolides inhibit platelet-activating factor (PAF). PAF, produced by a variety of tissues, not only induces aggregation of the blood platelets, it also causes bronchoconstriction, cutaneous vasodilation, chemotaxis of phagocytes, hypotension, and the release of inflammatory compounds, such as enzymes and oxidants, from phagocytes.[23] In short, it mimics many of the features seen in allergic response. All of these actions of PAF are blocked by the ginkgolides, particularly ginkgolide B. Possibly the ginkgolides' most significant effect is an increase in blood fluidity, thereby improving circulation. Bilobalide acts in concert with the ginkgolides to improve the tolerance of brain tissue to hypoxia and to increase cerebral circulation.

Federal health authorities in Germany have declared GBE to be an effective treatment for cerebral circulatory disturbances resulting in reduced functional capacity and vigilance. Some of the symptoms resulting from such disturbances are vertigo, tinnitus, weakened memory, and mood swings accompanied by anxiety. These authorities have also found the extract useful for the treatment of certain other types of peripheral vascular disease, specifically, the peripheral arterial circulatory disturbance known as intermittent claudication. This condition, caused by sclerosis of the arteries of the leg, is characterized by a constant or cramping pain in the calf muscles brought on by walking a short distance. It is not uncommon among older persons and apparently responds well, at least in the initial stages, to treatment with GBE.[22]

Side effects of GBE administration are neither numerous nor frequent. They may include gastrointestinal disturbances, headache, and allergic skin reactions.

Although the extract is sold in Europe as an approved drug and is available there in a variety of dosage forms including tablets, liquids, and parenteral preparations for intravenous administration, it is not an approved drug in the United States. GBE is sold here as a food supplement, usually in the form of tablets containing 40 mg. of the extract. Recommended dosage is 1 tablet 3 times daily with meals. Practically all of the scientific and clinical research on GBE has been carried out with an extract designated EGb 761 produced in Germany by the Dr. Willmar Schwabe GmbH & Co. or its subsidiaries. The bioequivalence of other GBE products has not been demonstrated.

Other Peripheral Arterial Circulatory Disorders

The use of ginkgo leaf extract (GBE) for the treatment of intermittent claudication has already been discussed. Father Sebastian Kneipp, a well-known German folk-healer of the nineteenth century, recommended both **Rosemary** leaves (*Rosmarinus officinalis* L., family Lamiaceae) and their contained volatile oil for their tonic effect on circulation. Taken internally or applied externally, often in the form of a bath, rosemary oil has been said to improve chronic circulatory weakness, including hypotension.[24]

Hänsel has noted that the internal use of rosemary for this purpose is still controversial.[25] While external use might result in some slight increase in blood flow in the cutaneous vasculature as a result of the oil's counterirritant properties, it is difficult to see how this might produce any substantial improvement in peripheral circulation. Rosemary cannot be recommended for this purpose at this time. It does possess some carminative properties and may be useful as a treatment for indigestion.

Venous Disorders

Varicose Vein Syndrome

Disorders of the veins most amenable to herbal therapy are those associated with varicosities. These are characterized by abnormally dilated, tortuous, readily visible, usually superficial veins, primarily of the extremities. The condition is often associated with aching discomfort or pain, depending on its severity and the presence of thrombus-associated inflammation, loss of endothelium, and edema.[26]

It is now recognized that varicose vein syndrome is largely the result of the action of lysosomal enzymes that destroy the network of proteoglycans in the elastic tissue of the veins. This facilitates the passage of electrolytes, proteins, and water through the venous walls, thereby producing edema. The enzymes also act not only to reduce the strength of the vessel walls but to cause them to dilate as well. The result is valvular incompetence, the blood flow tends to stagnate, and complications including thrombophlebitis may develop.[27]

Therapy for varicose vein syndrome has as its objectives:

1. Relief of existing edema,
2. Prevention of edema by reducing vessel permeability,
3. Reduction of blood stasis by increasing venous tonus,
4. Inhibition of the action of lysosomal enzymes, and
5. Neutralization of inflammatory and sclerotic processes.

In this connection, it must be noted that herbal treatment of varicose veins should not be expected to reverse changes in organic structures that have resulted from years of chronic varicosity. It may, however, provide some relief from the unpleasant symptoms by increasing capillary resistance, improving venous tonus, and even inhibiting the action of lysosomal enzymes.

Most of the phytomedicinals used to treat varicose vein syndrome are isolated chemicals or mixtures thereof, such as rutin, hesperidin, diosmin, coumarin, and the like. These will not be discussed here. By far the most effective plant drug employed for the disorder is:

Horse Chestnut Seed

The large, nearly globular, brown seeds of *Aesculus hippocastanum* L. (family Hippocastanaceae), or of closely related species, such as the American horse chestnut or Ohio buckeye, *A. glabra* Willd., are probably known to every schoolchild, being widely used in children's games. Superstitious adults in many countries carry them in their pockets to prevent or to cure arthritis and rheumatism. Because of their attractive red, yellow, or white flower clusters, the relatively large trees that bear them are widely cultivated.

Horse chestnut seeds contain a complex mixture of triterpenoid saponin glycosides designated aescin. This may be fractionated into an easily crystallizable mixture known as β-aescin and water-soluble components referred to as α-aescin. Flavonoids, including quercetin and kaempferol, are also present in the seed.[28]

Aescin has the ability to reduce lysosomal enzyme activity as much as 30 percent, apparently by stabilizing the cholesterol-containing membranes of the lysosomes and limiting release of the enzymes. The compound also restricts edema by reducing the transcapillary filtration of water and protein. It has some beneficial diuretic effect as well. In addition, it has been shown to increase the tonus of the veins, thus improving return blood flow to the heart.[27] As can be seen from the earlier discussion, all of these actions would prove beneficial for the treatment of varicose veins.

Horse chestnut seeds are normally utilized in the form of an aqueous-alcoholic extract that is dried and adjusted to a uniform concentration of 16 to 21 percent triterpene glycosides, calculated as aescin. Initial oral dosage is equivalent to 90 to 150 mg. of aescin, but following improvement, this may be reduced to 35 to 70 mg. daily. As of this writing, standardized horse chestnut extracts or dosage forms prepared from them are not commercially available in the United States. Extemporaneous preparation of a hydroalcoholic extract is possible, but standardization is difficult.

A number of ointments and liniments containing horse chestnut extract are available in Europe. Some of these are endorsed by the manufacturers, not only for local application to superficial varicose veins but for the treatment of hemorrhoids as well. Since evidence regarding the transdermal absorption of aescin is lacking and because hemorrhoids are related to both arterial and venous circulation, the efficacy of such preparations, particularly in the treatment of hemorrhoids, is doubtful.[29] Neither horse chestnut extract nor its contained aescin is recognized by the FDA in this country as an effective ingredient in hemorrhoid preparations.

German Commission E has approved the use of horse chestnut seeds for the treatment of chronic venous insufficiency of various origins as well as pain and a feeling of heaviness in the legs. It is also recommended for varicose veins and postthrombotic syndrome. The herb is antiexudative and acts to increase tonus of the veins. Side effects are uncommon, but gastrointestinal irritation may occur.[30] Isolated cases of renal and hepatic toxicity as well as anaphylactic reactions have been reported following intravenous administration, but these appear to be exceptional.[31]

Butcher's-Broom

The rhizome and roots of *Ruscus aculeatus* L., a fairly common, short evergreen shrub of the family Liliaceae, has acquired some reputation recently as a useful treatment of varicose vein syndrome. Much less studied, both chemically and clinically, than horse chestnut, the herb contains a mixture of steroidal saponins, particularly the modified cholesterol derivatives ruscogenin and neoruscogenin. These are said to exert anti-inflammatory effects and to increase the tonus of the veins.[32]

In Europe, the herb is available in capsules or tablets containing about 300 mg. each of a dried extract. Ointments and suppositories for the treatment of hemorrhoids are also available.[33] Butcher's-broom capsules are available in the United States. Although toxicity has not been reported, much additional work must be carried out before the efficacy of butcher's-broom can be established with certainty.

REFERENCE NOTES

1. Covinsky, J.O. and Willett, M.S.: "Chapter 11" in *Pharmacotherapy: A Pathophysiologic Approach*, J.T. DiPiro, R.L. Talbert, P.E. Hayes, G.C. Yee, and L. M. Posey, eds., Elsevier, New York, 1989, p. 115.

2. Hänsel, R.: *Phytopharmaka*, 2nd ed., Springer-Verlag, Berlin, 1991, pp. 25-40.

3. Tyler, V.E., Brady, L.R., and Robbers, J.E.: *Pharmacognosy*, 9th ed., Lea & Febiger, Philadelphia, 1988, pp. 171-173.

4. Gross, G.J.: "Chapter 24" in *Modern Pharmacology*, 3rd ed., C.R. Craig and R. E. Stitzel, eds., Little, Brown, Boston, 1990, pp. 322-332.

5. Haas, H.: *Arzneipflanzenkunde*, B.I. Wissenschaftsverlag, Mannheim, 1991, pp. 13-17.

6. Hamon, N.W.: *Canadian Pharmaceutical Journal* **121**:708-709, 724 (1988).

7. *Bundesanzeiger* (Cologne, Germany): January 3, 1984; May 5, 1988.

8. Tierney, L.M., Jr. and Erskine, J.M.: "Chapter 9" in *Current Medical Diagnosis and Treatment 1990*, S. A. Schroeder, M.A. Krupp, L.M. Tierney, Jr., and S. J. McPhee, Appleton & Lange, Norwalk, Connecticut, 1990, p. 301.

9. Foster, S.: *Garlic: Allium sativum*, Botanical Series No. 311, American Botanical Council, Austin, Texas, 1991, 7 pp.

10. Kleijnen, J., Knipschild, P., and Ter Riet, G.: *British Journal of Clinical Pharmacology* **28**:535-544 (1989).

11. Mader, F.H.: *Arzneimittel-Forschung* **40(II)**: 1111-1116 (1990).

12. Friedl, C.: *Zeitschrift für Phytotherapie* **11**: 203 (1990).

13. Lawson, L.D., and Hughes, B.G.: *Planta Medica* **58**:345-350 (1992).

14. Lawson, L.D., Wang, Z.-Y.J., and Hughes, B.G.: *Planta Medica* **57**:363-370 (1991).

15. Anon.: *Deutsche Apotheker Zeitung* **132**:643-644 (1992).

16. Reuter, H.D.: *Deutsche Apotheker Zeitung* **12**:83-91 (1991).

17. *Bundesanzeiger* (Cologne, Germany): July 6, 1988.

18. Quandt, C.M.: "Chapter 17" in *Pharmacotherapy: A Pathophysiologic Approach*, J.T. DiPiro, R.L. Talbert, P.E. Hayes, G.C. Yee, and L.M Posey, eds., Elsevier, New York, 1989, p. 271.

19. Bradberry, J.C.: "Chapter 18" in *Pharmacotherapy: A Pathophysiologic Approach*, J.T. DiPiro, R.L. Talbert, P.E. Hayes, G.C. Yee, and L.M. Posey, eds., Elsevier, New York, 1989, p. 280.

20. Tyler, V.E.: *Nutrition Forum* **8**:23 (1991).

21. Del Tredici, P.: *Arnoldia* **51**:2-15 (1991).

22. Hänsel, R.: *Phytopharmaka*, 2nd ed., Springer-Verlag, Berlin, 1991, pp. 59-72.

23. Brestel, E.P. and Van Dyke, K.: "Chapter 42" in *Modern Pharmacology*, 3rd ed., C.R. Craig and R.E. Stitzel, eds., Little, Brown, Boston, 1991, pp. 567-569.

24. Weiss, R.F.: *Herbal Medicine*, AB Arcanum, Gothenburg, Sweden, 1988, pp. 185-186.

25. Hänsel, R.: *Phytopharmaka*, 2nd ed., Springer-Verlag, Berlin, 1991, p. 55.

26. Tierney, L.M., Jr. and Erskine, J.M.: "Chapter 9" in *Current Medical Diagnosis and Treatment 1990*, S.A. Schroeder, M.A. Krupp, L.M. Tierney, Jr., and S.J. McPhee, Appleton & Lange, Norwalk, Connecticut, 1990, p. 317.

27. Haas, H.: *Arzneipflanzenkunde*, B.I. Wissenschaftsverlag, Mannheim, 1991, pp. 31-40.

28. Braun, H. and Frohne, D.: *Heilpflanzen-Lexikon für Ärzte und Apotheker*, Gustav Fischer Verlag, Stuttgart, 1987, pp. 7-9.

29. Weiss, R.F.: *Herbal Medicine*, AB Arcanum, Gothenburg, Sweden, 1988, p. 187.

30. *Bundesanzeiger* (Cologne, Germany): December 5, 1984.

31. Vogel, G.: *Zeitschrift für Phytotherapie* **10**:102-106 (1989).

32. Müller, I.: *Deutsche Apotheker Zeitung* **113**:1370-1375 (1973).

33. Braun, H. and Frohne, D.: *Heilpflanzen-Lexikon für Ärzte und Apotheker*, Gustav Fischer Verlag, Stuttgart, 1987, pp. 212-213.

Chapter 8

Nervous System Disorders

ANXIETY AND SLEEP DISORDERS

Anxiety is apprehension, tension, or uneasiness that stems from external stress or from no apparent cause. It is usually a normal response, but when it becomes disproportionate to the causal stimulus, or when no stimulus can be identified, it becomes disruptive.[1] Insomnia, the inability to attain restful sleep in adequate amounts, is often a transient response to the anxiety produced by stressful situations. It may also be symptomatic of more serious physiologic or psychologic conditions or the use of various drugs, including alcohol.[2]

Anxiety and insomnia are amenable to treatment with drugs that exert a depressant effect on the central nervous system (CNS). In many cases, the same CNS depressants are used to treat both conditions; however, a larger dose is customarily employed to induce sleep. The agents used are referred to by a number of names, including sleep aids, sedatives, hypnotics, soporifics, antianxiety agents, anxiolytics, calmatives, and minor tranquilizers. All of these terms are more or less synonymous, although, as noted, the degree of response obtained is dose-dependent. Most of the prescription drugs in these categories involve some risk of overdose, tolerance, habituation, and addiction.[3]

The herbs commonly used for their sedative effects do not suffer these drawbacks, but neither do they possess the degree of activity shown by the prescription drugs. In fact, the action of many traditional plant hypnotics is so slight as to remain uncertain.

Valerian

Probably the most effective of the entire group is valerian. The dried rhizome and roots of a tall perennial herb, *Valeriana officinalis*

L. (family Valerianaceae), have enjoyed a considerable reputation as a minor tranquilizer and sleep aid for more than 1,000 years. They contain from 0.3 to 0.7 percent of an unpleasant-smelling volatile oil containing bornyl acetate and the sesquiterpene derivatives valerenic acid and acetoxyvalerenic acid. Also present is 0.5 to 2 percent of a mixture of lipophilic iridoid principles known as valepotriates. These monocyclic monoterpenes are quite unstable and occur only in the fresh plant material or in that dried at temperatures under 40° C. In addition, various sugars, amino acids, free fatty acids, and aromatic acids have been isolated from the drug.[4]

Identity of the active principles of valerian has been a subject of controversy for many years. Initially, the calmative effect was attributed to the volatile oil; indeed, this kind of activity was long associated with most herbs containing oils with disagreeable odors. Then, beginning in 1966 with the isolation of the valepotriates, the property was attributed to them for a 20-year period. This was done in spite of the fact that they were highly unstable and were contained in most valerian preparations only in small amounts. Finally, in 1988, Krieglstein and Grusla showed that although valerian did produce CNS depression, neither the tested valepotriates, nor the sesquiterpenes valerenic acid or valeranone, nor the volatile oil itself displayed any such effect in rats.[5] Although the active principles of valerian remain unidentified, it seems possible that a combination of volatile oil, valepotriates, and possibly certain water-soluble constituents may be involved.

Because the valepotriates possess an epoxide structure, they demonstrate alkylating activity in cell cultures. This caused concern that the herb might possess potential toxicity. However, those valepotriates decompose rapidly in the stored drug and also are not readily absorbed. For these reasons, no toxicity has ever been demonstrated in intact animals or human beings, so there is no cause for concern.

Both Hänsel and Foster have reviewed a number of the recent clinical investigations demonstrating the effectiveness of valerian as a sleep aid and minor tranquilizer.[4,6] Based on the generally favorable results of these and other studies, the German Commission E has approved valerian as a calmative and sleep-promoting agent useful in treating states of unrest and anxiety-produced sleep disturbances.[7]

The herb may be administered several times daily as a tea prepared from 2 to 3 g. (1 teaspoonful) of the dried rhizome and roots. Equivalent amounts (1/2-1 teaspoonful or 3-5 ml.) of a tincture or extract may also be employed. Valerian is also used externally in the form of a calmative bath (100 g. per tub of water), but evidence supporting its effectiveness by this route is much less substantial. In the preparation of any of these dosage forms, the use of fresh or recently and carefully dried (temperatures under 40° C) herb is most likely to yield satisfactory results. Side effects and contraindications to the use of valerian have not been reported.

Passion Flower

A 1986 survey of herbal sedatives in Britain revealed that the most popular, based on its incorporation in the largest number of proprietary preparations, was passion flower.[8] Consisting of the dried flowering and fruiting top of a perennial climbing vine, *Passiflora incarnata* L. (family Passifloraceae), passion flower is, in spite of its popularity, a relatively unproven minor tranquilizer. Its principal constituents include up to 2.5 percent flavonoids, especially vitexin, as well as coumarin, umbelliferone, and 0.05 percent maltol. Harmala-type indole alkaloids, including harman, harmine, harmaline, and harmalol are present in small amounts (up to 0.01 percent).[9]

Administered intraperitoneally to rats, passion flower extract significantly prolonged sleeping time and affected locomotor activity. These and related activities could not be attributed to either the flavonoids or the alkaloids in the extract.[10] Clinical studies are required to verify such activity in human beings.

In 1978, the FDA prohibited the use of passion flower in OTC sedative preparations on the grounds that it had not been proven safe and effective.[11] The German Commission E, however, has authorized its use in the treatment of nervous unrest, citing its ability to bring about a reduction in mobility in animal experiments.[12] The usual daily dose is 4 to 8 g. (3-6 teaspoonfuls) taken as a tea in divided doses. Side effects and contraindications have not been reported.

Hops

Another popular herbal sleep aid is hops, the dried strobile with its glandular trichomes of *Humulus lupulus* L., family Cannabidaceae. The herb contains about 15 to 30 percent of a resin which accounts for its bitter taste and for its well-established use as a preservative in the brewing of beer. On the other hand, the sedative properties of hops are not well-established, and much misinformation exists in the literature.

Hänsel and Wagener found that hop resin had no CNS depressant effect when taken orally.[13] However, when the herb is stored, bitter principles such as humulone and lupulone undergo auto-oxidation to produce a C_5-alcohol designated 2-methyl-3-buten-2-ol or, more simply, methylbutenol. A hops sample stored for two years contains about 0.04 percent methylbutenol. This volatile compound does produce CNS-depressant effects when inhaled, and this has been postulated to account for the soporific effects of hop-filled pillows. However, a single effective dose of methylbutenol would require all of the compound contained in 150 g. of hops.[14] It must be concluded that both the CNS-depressant activity and the identity of any active sedative principles in hop extracts or preparations are questionable at this time.

Catnip

The dried leaves and flowering tops of *Nepeta cataria* L., family Lamiaceae, have long been known to induce a kind of stimulation in cats that has become known as the catnip response.[15] In addition, the herb enjoys a substantial folkloric reputation as a calmative and sleep aid in humans.[16] In this regard, the effects of catnip closely parallel those of valerian, which also stimulates cats but sedates people. The 1969 report that catnip produced psychedelic effects in those smoking it was based on a confusion of the plant with cannabis.[17,18] Nevertheless, the misinformation continues to be quoted in the literature.

Scientific support for the sedative effect of catnip is insubstantial, being based on a series of papers involving the administration of various types of herbal extracts to chicks and observing their effects on sleep behavior.[19] A hot-water extract of catnip previously extracted with hexane to render it lactone-free was particularly effective. The chemical compounds responsible for catnip's sedative effects remain unidentified. A tea prepared from 1 to 2 teaspoonfuls (1-2 g.) of the herb per cup (240 ml.) continues to be widely used as a sleep aid. Side effects and contraindications have not been reported with normal use.[20] The herb is included in this work on the basis of its potential rather than its proven efficacy.

L-Tryptophan

Although not an herb, L-tryptophan is a natural amino acid that occurs in concentrations of 1 to 2 percent in many plant and animal proteins. It is produced in quantity by fermentation utilizing selected bacteria. L-Tryptophan is an essential amino acid that must be obtained from exogenous sources; the minimal daily requirement for an adult is 3 mg. ($\pm$ 30 percent) per kilogram of body weight. For a 180-lb. person this is equivalent to about 0.25 g.[21]

Studies have shown that 1-g. doses of L-tryptophan reduce sleep latency by increasing subjective "sleepiness" and also decrease waking time.[22] The amino acid functions by bringing about an increase in serotonin in certain brain cells, thus inducing sleep but also assisting in the treatment of pain, mental depression, and other behavioral conditions.[23] Although never approved as a drug, capsules and tablets of the amino acid in amounts ranging from 100 to 667 mg. were widely sold as sleep aids in health food stores until 1989.

In that year, cases of a serious blood disorder, eosinophilia-myalgia syndrome (EMS) began to occur in otherwise healthy individuals who had consumed quantities of L-tryptophan. The FDA ordered the recall of manufactured L-tryptophan in any form at all dosage levels, but the product had already caused 5,000 cases of EMS and 27 deaths.[24] Eventually all of the suspect amino acid was traced to a single manufacturer, Showa Denko K. K. in Japan. That organization had used a new genetically engineered bacterium to produce the L-tryptophan and had also modified the customary purification procedure. Suspicion regarding the cause of EMS then shifted away from the L-tryptophan to contaminants produced, or at least not removed, during the fermentation process. One contaminant has now been identified as 1,1'-ethylidenebis(L-tryptophan);[25]

another was found to be 3-phenyl-amino-L-aniline. The latter compound is similar to a contaminant in industrial rapeseed oil that was responsible for an outbreak of EMS in Spain in 1981 when the impure oil was used for culinary purposes.[26]

As of this writing, some uncertainties still remain about the ability of L-tryptophan manufacturers to produce a pure amino acid free of toxic contaminants. Consequently, the FDA has not yet authorized the sale of L-tryptophan. There certainly exists a need for additional research into the safety and efficacy of pure L-tryptophan as a potentially valuable therapeutic agent. Until the time when safety of the marketed product can be assured, the consumption of manufactured L-tryptophan in any form must be avoided.

DEPRESSION

Depression, the inability to experience pleasure or happiness, usually accompanied by feelings of helplessness and lack of self-worth, is one of the most common of the psychiatric disorders. It is a so-called affective disorder, meaning that it causes changes in emotions, feelings, or mental state. When it results from some severe emotional strain, such as loss of a loved one or self-pity brought about by a disease, the condition is usually self-limiting. In the absence of such an identifiable cause, it is known as endogenous depression, that is, depression originating from within.

Depending upon the exact type and severity of the depressed state, it may be treated in a variety of ways, including psychotherapy, electroshock, or the administration of drugs, particularly the tricyclic antidepressants or monoamine oxidase (MAO) inhibitors.

St. John's Wort

One of the most popular herbal remedies for depression is St. John's wort. A tea prepared from the leaves and flowering tops of *Hypericum perforatum* L. is widely used in Europe today for its antidepressive effects. It is viewed there as an alternative to the synthetic drugs, not only for the treatment of depression but for nervous unrest and sleep disturbances as well.[27]

Standard reference works attribute the antidepressive effects of St. John's wort to its content of hypericin, pseudohypericin, and related naphthodianthrones that are found in the herb to the extent of about 0.1 percent.[28] And, indeed, in-vitro tests carried out in 1984 confirmed that hypericin inhibited both type A and type B MAO.[29] More recent studies, however, have not been able to confirm this inhibition by hypericin but instead have identified plant fractions containing xanthones and flavonoids as being active MAO inhibitors.[30,31]

Although it is not possible at this time to identify with certainty the active antidepressant principle(s) in St. John's wort, it may be concluded that the herb is apparently modestly effective in this regard, probably due to contained MAO inhibitors. This activity has been demonstrated in small animals with an extract of the herb,[32] and initial clinical tests in humans have also shown antidepressive effects.[33]

Side effects were not noted in the latter study, but more recently the safety of St. John's wort was called into question when scientists demonstrated the cytotoxic and mutagenic nature of some extracts of it.[34] Concern over this potential carcinogenicity led to identification of quercetin, a common plant constituent, as the responsible compound. Quercetin is widely distributed in the plant kingdom. It is estimated that the average person consumes about 50 mg. of it and related flavonoids in fruits and vegetables daily, and use of an herb such as St. John's wort in normal amounts would increase this by about 1 mg. In view of this and of the considerable uncertainty about the carcinogenic properties of quercetin, Commission E of the German Federal Health Agency has noted that concern regarding its toxicity is unwarranted.[35]

Hypericin is known to be phototoxic in grazing animals, resulting in dermatitis of the skin and inflammation of the mucous membranes on exposure to direct sunlight.[36] Although a literature search failed to identify a single case involving humans, caution regarding exposure to bright sunlight is advised, particularly for fair-skinned persons or those with known photosensitivities.[37]

Like most herbs, St. John's wort is valued in folk medicine for a number of conditions unrelated to its principal antidepressant effects. The fresh flowers are crushed and macerated in olive oil which, after several weeks' standing in the sun, acquires a reddish color. This so-called red oil may be taken internally just like the tea, but it is more commonly applied locally to relieve inflammation and promote healing.

In recent studies, both hypericin and the closely related pseudo-hypericin have been shown to exhibit antiviral effects in mice infected experimentally with two murine leukemia retroviruses.[38] This, of course, raises the possibility that these compounds from St. John's wort might prove useful in the treatment of AIDS- and HIV-infected patients. Additional studies are certainly warranted and, in fact, are now in progress.[39]

Preparation of tea from this plant involves pouring 1 cup (240 ml.) of boiling water over 1 to 2 heaping teaspoonfuls (2-4 g.) of the herb and allowing it to steep for about 10 minutes. Because the active antidepressant principles remain unidentified, it is not possible to calculate the quantity that would be present in such a preparation. St. John's wort is said to be most effective when 1 to 2 cups (240-480 ml.) of the tea are consumed daily over an extended period of time (4-6 weeks).

PAIN (GENERAL)

Pain is an unpleasant sensory experience associated with actual or potential tissue damage. It may be acute or chronic in character; both types are customarily treated by the administration of drugs known as analgesics. The analgesics used to treat pain are often classified into two categories: the narcotics that bind to opioid receptors, and the non-narcotics that lack an affinity for such receptors.[40] Although the most effective herbal analgesics, e.g., morphine and codeine, fall into the first category, they will not be discussed here because they are not available without a prescription. The action of the latter type is peripheral and, in the case of the salicylates, apparently results from the inhibition of prostaglandin synthesis.

Willow Bark

Among the non-narcotics used to treat pain, the salicylates are probably the most common. Certain salicylate derivatives occur in herbs, particularly in willow bark. Use of the bark of *Salix alba* L. and related *Salix* species for their analgesic and anti-inflammatory properties will be discussed in detail in Chapter 10, "Arthritic and Musculoskeletal Disorders." It is sufficient to say here that the active principle, salicin, occurs in the herb in such small amounts as to render its use as a painkiller impractical. Somewhere between 3 and 21 cups (0.75-5 liters) of willow bark tea would have to be consumed to obtain a single average dose. In view of the high tannin content of the bark, this is impractical.

Capsicum

Variously know as red pepper, cayenne pepper, and chili pepper, the herb consists of the dried ripe fruit of *Capsicum frutescens* L., *C. annuum* L. and a large number of varieties and hybrids of these members of the family Solanaceae. The medicinal value of capsicum is directly related to its pungency. This varies greatly according to the specific variety involved and its content of capsaicin. Normally this phenolic derivative occurs in the fruit in concentrations of about 0.02 percent. Its presence accounts for the long-standing folk usage of capsicum as a counterirritant in medicine and a condiment in the culinary arts.[41]

During the past decade, creams containing low concentrations (0.025-0.075 percent) of capsaicin have been found to be effective in the treatment of intractable pain such as that associated with herpes zoster (shingles), postmastectomy and postamputation neuroma (phantom pain syndrome), diabetic neuropathy, and even cluster headache. The compound causes a depletion of substance P, a neuropeptide that mediates the transmission of pain impulses from the peripheral nerves to the spinal cord. So even if the condition causing the pain continues to be present, no perception of it reaches the brain.[42] Depletion of substance P does not occur immediately. Effective use of the cream requires topical application 4 or 5 times daily for a period of at least 4 weeks. Users must be especially careful to wash their hands thoroughly after each application and to avoid touching the eyes or mucous membranes after applying the product.[43] A phytomedicine containing 0.075 percent capsaicin in a cream base has been approved by the FDA for OTC sale.

HEADACHE

Headache, a condition experienced by about 15 percent of the population on a weekly basis, usually is a symptom of an underlying disorder. Almost all of them are vascular in character or are produced by tension (muscle contraction) or a combination of the two types. A small percentage results from underlying intracranial, systemic, or psychologic conditions. Migraine is a type of throbbing vascular headache that affects about 10 percent of Americans, mostly females.[44] A variant vascular headache is cluster, which recurs episodically at intervals of months to years. Its victims are primarily male.

Antimigraine Herbs

Treatment of vascular headache involves not only relief of the intense pain of an acute attack but also the prevention (prophylaxis) of additional attacks. During the past decade, research has demonstrated the prophylactic value in migraine treatment of the following herb.

Feverfew

Valued since the time of Dioscorides (78 A.D.) as a febrifuge (antipyretic), the leaves of *Tanacetum parthenium* (L.) Schultz Bip. have now been shown to be useful in reducing the frequency and severity of migraine as well as the discomfort of the frequently associated nausea and vomiting. A number of clinical trials have verified the utility of relatively small amounts (ca. 60-82 mg.) of the carefully dried leaves in preventing such attacks.[45]

The principle that is primarily responsible for this effect is parthenolide, a sesquiterpene lactone whose concentration varies widely in different feverfew samples. Canadian authorities have recommended that a quality feverfew should contain a minimum concentration of 0.2 percent parthenolide. Parthenolide, and possibly some of the related sesquiterpene lactones that accompany it in feverfew, apparently act as serotonin antagonists tending to inhibit the release of that compound from blood platelets. Serotonin (5-HT) is the most important vasoactive amine mediating vascular headache.[46] It also acts to lower the pain threshold.

Feverfew is commonly consumed simply by chewing the fresh leaves of the plant or those that have been freeze-dried or heat-dried at a relatively low temperature (37° C). This practice results in minor ulcerations of the oral mucosa in about 12 percent of the patients, and irritation of tongue and oral mucosa accompanied by swelling of the lips in 7 percent of the consumers. These conditions require administration of the plant to be discontinued.[47]

Feverfew tablets or capsules are available commercially, each usually containing at least 300 mg. of the herb. Manufacturers commonly recommend consumption of 2 to 6 dosage units daily. If the feverfew is of good quality, this is a much larger dose than is actually required for migraine prophylaxis. A quantity containing 250 μg. of parthenolide is now considered an adequate daily dose. At the 0.2 percent minimum quality standard, this would amount to 125 mg. of herb, less than 1 tablet or capsule daily. However, in view of the variable quality of British feverfew herb and its preparations and the extremely poor quality of the North American product, it may be necessary to utilize this quantity of the substandard material to receive a therapeutic dose.[48,49,50] But even then, therapeutic efficacy is not assured. No parthenolide could be detected in two out of three feverfew products purchased in Louisiana health food stores.[51] Whether this is due to the use of plant material from different chemotypes, or to adulteration or substitution, is unknown. Standardization of the herbal material on the basis of its parthenolide content is urgently required if this potentially valuable herb is to be used effectively.

Caffeine-Containing Beverages

These CNS-stimulant plant products are most commonly employed simply to overcome drowsiness, but in addition, they are used therapeutically as adjuncts in the treatment of headache. The acute consumption of caffeine in conjunction with OTC analgesics such as aspirin or acetaminophen increases their activity by as much as 40 percent, depending on the specific type of pain involved. This beneficial effect is apparently due to the ability of caffeine to cause constriction of the cerebral blood vessels and, possibly, to facilitate the absorption of other drugs. The enhancement is short-lived, diminishing greatly on repeated (chronic) co-administration.

The principal caffeine beverages are prepared from:

Coffee–dried ripe seed of *Coffea arabica* L. (family Rubiaceae);

Tea–leaves and leaf buds of *Camellia sinensis* (L.) O. Kuntze (family Theaceae);

Kola (Cola)–dried cotyledon of *Cola nitida* (Vent.) Schott & Endl. and other *Cola* spp. (family Sterculiaceae);

Cacao (Cocoa)–roasted seed of *Theobroma cacao* L. (family Sterculiaceae);

Guarana–crushed seed of *Paullinia cupana* H.B.K. (family Sapindaceae); and

Maté–dried leaves of *Ilex paraguariensis* St.-Hil. (family Aquifoliaceae).

Depending on its exact mode of preparation, 1 cup (240 ml.) of beverage prepared from these herbs will contain amounts of caffeine ranging from about 10 mg. for cocoa to some 30 mg. for tea to approximately 100 mg. for coffee. So-called cola-flavored carbonated beverages are prepared using only minute amounts of cola. They do contain about 50 mg. per bottle of caffeine, which is added as a "flavor." In this country, caffeine is also added to a variety of food products, including baked goods, frozen dairy desserts, gelatin puddings, soft candy, and the like.[52]

Caffeine-containing beverages are used in combination with salicylates for the treatment of headache or with ergot alkaloids (ergotamine) for migraine. The customary dose is a quantity equivalent to 100-200 mg. of caffeine.[53]

It should also be noted that caffeine and the other naturally occurring xanthine derivatives, theobromine and theophylline, possess a diuretic action, but it is relatively weak and of short duration. Neither caffeine nor any of the various beverages containing it is extensively used for this purpose because tachyphylaxis develops rapidly on continued administration–a frequent situation with such drinks–and diuretic effectiveness is greatly diminished.

TOOTHACHE

Tooth pain usually results from a pathologic condition of the dentin, the pulp, or the supporting periodontum. The manifestations most amenable to temporary treatment with phytomedicinal agents are those resulting from caries or fractures. Either of these events results in an exposure of the dentin which, when subjected to heat, cold, or pressure, stimulates the numerous free nerve endings in the pulp, resulting in pain. If the pulp itself is exposed, the ache is continuous; if the pulp becomes infected, the pain will also be severe.[54]

The proper recourse for any toothache is timely treatment by a qualified dentist. This might consist of filling, root canal therapy, extraction, periodontal treatment, or the like. However, if professional care is not available, the pain may be allayed by the temporary use of appropriate herbal remedies. Such action must be viewed as only an emergency measure because prolonged use of self-selected remedies may exacerbate the underlying condition causing the pain.

Clove Oil

Probably the best-known herbal product used to obtain transient relief from toothache is clove oil. This is obtained by steam distillation from clove (cloves), the dried flower-buds of *Syzgium aromaticum* (L.) Merr. & T.M. Perry of the family Myrtaceae. For many years, the correct scientific name of the plant was considered to be either *Eugenia caryophyllata* Thunb. or *Caryophyllus aromaticus* L. These names are still encountered in the older herbal literature. All three designations refer to the same species. Clove of good quality yields about 15 to 25 percent of a volatile oil that has both local analgesic and antiseptic properties. These are due to a number of phenolic substances contained in the oil, the principal one of which is eugenol, comprising about 85 percent of the total.

Although clove oil is sufficiently irritating to preclude general internal usage, it has long been employed as a local analgesic or obtundent for the relief of toothache. Eugenol, like other phenols, acts on contact to depress sensory receptors involved in pain perception. The mechanism of action involves, in part, a pronounced inhibition of prostaglandin biosynthesis resulting from blockages of both the cyclooxygenase and lipoxygenase metabolic pathways.[55] In practice, a pledget of cotton is dipped in the undiluted oil and applied to the surface of the aching tooth and surrounding tissue, or if possible, inserted directly into the cavity where it will alleviate the pain for several hours. The oil is also used in mouthwashes, in concentrations of 1 to 5 percent, for its antiseptic effects.

Various forms of clove (actually listed as cloves), including the volatile oil, appear as safe food additives on the GRAS list of the Food and Drug Administration. The American Dental Association has accepted clove oil, or its constituent eugenol, for professional use only, not for nonprescription use. In Germany, Commission E has approved the use of clove oil as a local anesthetic and antiseptic.[56]

Prickly Ash Bark

The barks of two species of *Zanthoxylum* are used more or less interchangeably as toothache remedies in this country. Both *Z. americanum* Mill., the northern prickly ash, and *Z. clava-herculis* L., the southern prickly ash, are sometimes referred to as toothache trees. These members of the family Rutaceae both yield prickly barks that, on chewing, produce a tingling sensation in the mouth and are also effective remedies for toothache. For all practical purposes, the barks of the two species may be considered as a single herb. It was valued by the American Indians who chewed the bark and then packed the masticated quid around the ailing tooth to relieve the pain.[57]

Although prickly ash bark, under the title Xanthoxylum, held official status in the *USP* and then the *NF* from 1820 to 1947 and was employed as a diaphoretic and antirheumatic, the principle(s) responsible for its local anesthetic effect appear not to have been investigated scientifically. Older sources simply attribute the bark's pungency on chewing to its resin content.[58] More recent studies on a related West African species, *Z. zanthoxyloides* (Lam.) Watson, which has similar properties, associate at least some of its anti-inflammatory action with the presence of fagaramide, an aromatic acid amide. Fagaramide apparently acts as an inhibitor of prostaglandin synthesis and might account for some of the analgesic effects of the bark as well.[59] It is not known if the American *Zanthoxylum* species contain fagaramide.

Prickly ash bark is used for toothache today in the same manner as it was employed long ago by the American Indians. A small amount of the bark is chewed, and the moist mass is packed around the painful tooth as an emergency method of relieving pain. Adverse effects have not been reported from short-term use.

SEXUAL IMPOTENCE

The inability of a male to attain or maintain penile erection sufficient to complete intercourse is termed erectile dysfunction or, more commonly, impotence. Psychogenic factors such as sexual anxieties, guilt, fear, feelings of inadequacy, and the like, are responsible for 50 to 60 percent of erectile dysfunction. The remainder of such cases are caused by organic factors.[60]

Yohimbe

An herb that holds some promise in the treatment of erectile disfunction is yohimbe. Consisting of the bark of the West African tree *Pausinystalia yohimbe* (K. Schum.) Pierre of the family Rubiaceae, yohimbe contains about 6 percent of a mixture of alkaloids, the principal one of which is yohimbine. Both yohimbe and yohimbine have long enjoyed considerable reputations as aphrodisiacs.

Recent clinical studies have confirmed the value of yohimbine in treating impotence in human males. Some 46 percent of a group of patients being treated for psychogenic impotence reported a positive response to the drug, and 43 percent of patients with organic causes of impotence reported improvement in erectile function. Although questions remain regarding the action of yohimbine in the body, Reid and colleagues conclude that the alkaloid is a safe treatment for psychogenic impotence and is as effective as other modalities.[61] Tablets containing 5.4 mg. of yohimbine hydrochloride are currently being marketed.

In spite of this generally favorable information, yohimbe and yohimbine cannot be recommended for self-treatment. Neither is an approved drug for OTC sale in the United States, and the German Commission E does not recommend their therapeutic use. The Commission notes that there exists insufficient proof of their activity as well as an unacceptably high risk-benefit ratio. Side effects include agitation, tremors, insomnia, anxiety, hypertension, tachycardia, nausea, and vomiting.[62] In spite of this ruling, a large number of aphrodisiac preparations containing yohimbine continue to be marketed in Germany.

Ginkgo

The reports that prolonged oral administration of ginkgo biloba extract (see Chapter 7) may benefit persons suffering from erectile dysfunction are highly preliminary.[63] Additional data are required to support the possible use of GBE for this purpose.

REFERENCE NOTES

1. *Drug Evaluations*, 6th ed., American Medical Association, Chicago, 1986, pp. 81-84.

2. Caro, J. P. and Dombrowski, S.R.: "Chapter 10" in *Handbook of Nonprescription Drugs*, 9th ed., American Pharmaceutical Association, Washington, D.C., 1990, pp. 225-229.

3. *The Merck Manual of Diagnosis and Therapy*, 15th ed., Merck Sharp & Dohme Research Laboratories, Rahway, N.J., 1987, p. 1377.

4. Hänsel, R.: *Phytopharmaka*, 2nd ed., Springer-Verlag, Berlin, 1991, pp. 252-259.

5. Krieglstein, J. and Grusla, D.: *Deutsche Apotheker Zeitung* **128**:2041-2046 (1988).

6. Foster, S.: *Valerian:* Valeriana officinalis, Botanical Series No. 312, American Botanical Council, Austin, Texas, 1990, 8 pp.

7. *Bundesanzeiger* (Cologne, Germany): May 15, 1985; March 6, 1990.

8. Ross, M.S.F. and Anderson, L.A.: *International Journal of Crude Drug Research* **24**:1-6 (1986).

9. *Lawrence Review of Natural Products:* May, 1989.

10. Speroni, E. and Minghetti, A.: *Planta Medica* **54**:488-491 (1988).

11. *Federal Register* **43**(114):25578 (1978).

12. *Bundesanzeiger* (Cologne, Germany): November 30, 1985; March 6, 1990.

13. Hänsel, R. and Wagener, H.H.: *Arzneimittel-Forschung* **17**:79-81 (1967).

14. Hölzl, J.: *Zeitschrift für Phytotherapie* **13**:155-161 (1992).

15. Tucker, A.O. and Tucker, S. S.: *Economic Botany* **42**:214-231 (1988).

16. Tyler, V.E.: *Hoosier Home Remedies*, Purdue University Press, West Lafayette, Indiana, 1985, pp. 113-115.

17. Jackson, B. and Reed, A.: *Journal of the American Medical Association* **207**:1349-1350 (1969).

18. Poundstone, J.: *Journal of the American Medical Association* **208**:360 (1969).

19. Sherry, C.J. and Mitchell, J.P.: *International Journal of Crude Drug Research* **21**:89-92 (1983).

20. *Lawrence Review of Natural Products:* January, 1991.

21. Lentner, C., ed.: *Geigy Scientific Tables*, vol. 1, Ciba-Geigy, Basle, 1981, p. 235.

22. Hartmann, E.: *The Sleeping Pill*, Yale University Press, New Haven, 1978, pp. 162-181.

23. Craig, C.R.: "Chapter 27" in *Modern Pharmacology*, 3rd ed., C.R. Craig and R.E. Stitzel, eds., Little, Brown, Boston, 1990, pp. 391-392.

24. Gelb, L.N., ed.: *FDA Drug Bulletin* **20**(1):2-3 (1990).

25. Smith, J.J., et al. (8 other authors): *Tetrahedron Letters* **32**:991-994 (1991).

26. Anon.: *Health Foods Business* **38**(11):10 (1992).

27. Pahlow, M.: *Deutsche Apotheker Zeitung* **42**:2059-2060 (1984).

28. Wichtl, M., ed.: *Teedrogen*, Wissenschaftliche Verlagsgesellschaft, Stuttgart, 1984, pp. 178-180.

29. Suzuki, O., Katsumata, Y., Oya, M., Bladt, S., and Wagner, H.: *Planta Medica* **50**:272-274 (1984).

30. Hölzl, J., Demisch, L., and Gollnik, B.: *Planta Medica* **55**:643 (1989).

31. Hölzl, J.: *Deutsche Apotheker Zeitung* **130**:367 (1990).

32. Okpanyi, S.N. and Weischer, M.L.: *Arzneimittel-Forschung* **37**(I):10-13 (1987).

33. Müldner, H. and Zöller, M.: *Arzneimittel-Forschung* **34**(II):918-920 (1984).

34. Poginsky, B., Westendorf, J., Prosenc, N., Kuppe, M., and Marquardt, H.: *Deutsche Apotheker Zeitung* **128**:1364-1366 (1988).

35. Kommission E des Bundesgesundheitsamtes: *Deutsche Apotheker Zeitung* **128**:1499 (1988).

36. Roth, L.: *Hypericum-Hypericin: Botanik, Inhaltsstoffe, Wirkung*, ecomed, Landsberg/Lech, Germany, 1990, pp. 135-138.

37. Hobbs, C.: *HerbalGram* No. 18/19: 24-33 (1989).

38. Muruelo, D., Lavie, G., and Lavie, D.: *Proceedings of the National Academy of Science, U.S.A.* **85**:5230-5234 (1988).

39. James, J.S.: *AIDS Treatment News* No. 117: 3 (1990).

40. *Drug Evaluations,* 6th ed., American Medical Association, Chicago, 1986, p. 53.

41. Tyler, V.E., Brady, L.R., and Robbers, J.E.: *Pharmacognosy*, 9th ed., Lea & Febiger, Philadelphia, 1988, pp. 148-150.

42. McCourt, R.: *Discover* **12**(8):48-52 (1991).

43. Gossel, T.A.: *U.S. Pharmacist* **15**(12):27-30 (1990).

44. *Professional Guide to Diseases*, 3rd ed., Springhouse, Springhouse, Pennsylvania, 1989, pp. 584-586.

45. Awang, D.V.C.: *HerbalGram* No. 29:34-36, 66 (1993).

46. Taylor, J.W. and Cleary, J.D.: "Chapter 44" in *Pharmacotherapy: A Pathophysiologic Approach*, J.T. DiPiro, R.L. Talbert, P.E. Hayes, G.C. Yee, and L.M. Posey, eds., Elsevier, New York, 1989, pp. 661-663.

47. Foster, S.: *Feverfew:* Tanacetum parthenium, Botanical Series No. 310, American Botanical Council, Austin, Texas, 1991, 8 pp.

48. Awang, D.V.C., Dawson, B.A., Kindack, D.G., Crompton, C.W., and Heptinstall, S.: *Journal of Natural Products* **54**:1516-1521 (1991).

49. Heptinstall, S. et al. (5 other authors): *Journal of Pharmacy and Pharmacology* **44**:391-395 (1992).

50. Marles, R.J. et al. (8 other authors): *Journal of Natural Products* **55**:1044-1056 (1992).

51. Casteñeda-Acosta, J., Fischer, N.H., and Vargas, D.: *Journal of Natural Products*, **56**:90-98 (1993).

52. Tyler, V.E.: *The Honest Herbal*, 3rd ed., Pharmaceutical Products Press, Binghamton, New York, 1993, pp. 69-72.

53. Haas, H.: *Arzneipflanzenkunde*, B.I. Wissenschaftsverlag, Mannheim, 1991, pp. 44-45.

54. Baker, K.A.: "Chapter 23" in *Handbook of Nonprescription Drugs*, 9th ed., American Pharmaceutical Association, Washington, D.C., 1990, pp. 653-687.

55. Deininger, R.: *Zeitschrift für Phytotherapie* **12**:205-212 (1991).

56. *Bundesanzeiger* (Cologne, Germany): November, 30, 1985.

57. Mizelle, R.: *Encounter with the Toothache Tree*, Carolina Banks Publishing, Kitty Hawk, North Carolina, 1986, 52 pp.

58. Osol, A. and Farrar, G.E., Jr.: *The Dispensatory of the United States of America*, 24th ed., J.B. Lippincott, Philadelphia, 1947, pp. 1650-1651.

59. Oliver-Bever, B.: *Medicinal Plants in Tropical West Africa*, Cambridge University Press, Cambridge, 1986, pp. 32-33, 205-206.

60. *Professional Guide to Diseases*, 3rd ed., Springhouse, Springhouse, Pennsylvania, 1989, pp. 974-976.

61. Reid, K. et al. (6 other authors): *Lancet* **II**: 421-423 (1987).

62. *Bundesanzeiger* (Cologne, Germany): August 14, 1987; February 1, 1990.

63. Anon.: *Sex Over 40* **10**(4):6-7 (1991).

Chapter 9

Metabolic and Endocrine Problems

GYNECOLOGICAL DISORDERS

These include a variety of conditions, such as menopausal symptoms, premenstrual syndrome including mastodynia, and dysmenorrhea. All are directly or indirectly related to imbalances or deficiencies in the production of female sex hormones or prostaglandins.

In the female menopause, the period following the complete cessation of menstruation, estrogen production drops to about 10 percent of its premenopausal levels and progesterone production drops to nearly zero. This results in various symptoms, four of which are more or less common: (1) vasomotor disorders (hot flashes), (2) urogenital atrophy, (3) osteoporosis, and (4) psychological disturbances. Administration of conjugated equine estrogens is the normal treatment for menopausal symptoms.[1]

Premenstrual syndrome (PMS) is characterized by certain emotional and physical symptoms as well as behavioral changes that occur during the premenstrual (luteal) phase of the menstrual cycle, and then disappear several days after the onset of menstruation. Its etiology is unknown. Some studies suggest that normal fluctuations in estrogen and progesterone trigger the symptoms by an unknown mechanism. Stress may play a role, and some women appear to be predisposed to PMS by various genetic, biologic, or psychologic factors.[2]

Primary dysmenorrhea, that is, painful menstruation in the absence of pelvic pathology, occurs with considerable frequency, particularly among adolescent females. Pain usually begins with, or just slightly before, the onset of menstrual flow and lasts for periods of up to two days, seldom longer. It has now been shown that this condition is associated with an increased production and concentration of prostaglandin in the endometrium during the luteal and menstrual phases of the cycle. This results in hypercontractility of uterine muscle during dysmenorrhea. Prostaglandin inhibitors have proven to be very effective in relieving the associated symptoms.[3]

Although true female sex hormones have not been identified in higher plants, some herbs apparently contain compounds that produce similar effects.

Black Cohosh

The dried rhizome and roots of *Cimicifuga racemosa* (L.) Nutt., family Ranunculaceae, is sometimes referred to as black snakeroot or as cimicifuga. It has an ancient reputation as a remedy for the treatment of "female complaints," a generic term that probably includes all of the gynecological disorders just discussed. As such, it was one of the ingredients in the famous proprietary medicine, Lydia E. Pinkham's Vegetable Compound.[4]

Hänsel has reviewed the literature supporting claims of estrogen-like activity for extracts of black cohosh.[5] A clinical study by Lehmann-Willenbrock and Riedel of hysterectomized patients with climacteric symptoms showed no significant differences among groups treated with various estrogens and those with black cohosh extracts.[6] The beneficial effects were slow to appear, requiring up to four weeks to reach a maximum. More recently, investigators have shown that an alcoholic extract of black cohosh suppressed hot flashes in menopausal women by reducing the secretion of luteinizing hormone (LH). It also suppressed LH production in ovariectomized rats. Three different synergistically acting compounds are thought to be responsible for this effect, but they remain unidentified.[7] The drug does contain a number of triterpenoid glycosides.

German Commission E has found black cohosh to be effective for the treatment of PMS and dysmenorrhea, as well as nervous conditions associated with menopause.[8] The herb is normally administered in the form of a 40 to 60 percent alcoholic extract in a quantity equivalent to 40 mg. of drug daily. A decoction prepared from 0.3 to 2.0 g. of the herb may also be employed. Administration of the drug sometimes causes stomach upsets; otherwise, no problems or contraindications have been reported. In view of the fact that no long-term toxicity studies on the use of black cohosh have been carried out, administration of the herb should be limited to a period of no longer than six months.

Chaste Tree Berry

The aromatic fruit of *Vitex agnus-castus* L., a small deciduous tree or large shrub of the family Verbenaceae that grows in the Mediterranean region, has long been used in European herbal medicine, but it is little known in the United States. In recent years, however, an extract of the fruit has become available in this country.[9]

Chaste tree berry is now believed to have dopaminergic properties; it thus inhibits the secretion of the peptide hormone prolactin by the pituitary gland.[5,10] Exactly what effect this has on PMS, dysmenorrhea, and menopause is not entirely clear, but it is known that amenorrhea is often associated with elevated blood levels of prolactin. Drugs that reduce prolactin concentrations usually restore the menstrual cycle to normal.[11] The nature of the chemical principle(s) in chaste tree berry responsible for this prolactin-depressant effect has not been established.

Although the German Commission E has recommended the use of chaste tree berry for a variety of menstrual disturbances,[12] Hänsel has suggested that its effectiveness for PMS and menopausal symptoms be reevaluated.[5] The herb is usually administered in the form of a concentrated alcoholic extract of the fruit; average dose is 20 mg. per day. Contraindications are not known, but use of the herb does occasionally produce an itchy rash in sensitive consumers.

Evening Primrose Oil

The small seed of this native American wildflower, *Oenothera biennis* L. (family Onagraceae), contains about 14 percent of a fixed oil of which 70 percent is *cis*-linolenic acid and 9 percent is *cis*-gamma-linolenic acid (GLA). The latter constituent is a relatively uncommon one, being found in quantity in only a few other plants, such as black currant and borage seeds.[13,14,15]

Theoretically, GLA can be converted directly to the prostaglandin precursor dihomo-GLA (DGLA), so administration of the oil containing it might be beneficial to persons unable to metabolize *cis*-linolenic acid to GLA and to produce subsequent intermediates of considerable metabolic significance, including prostaglandins.[16] Illnesses thought by some to arise from such metabolic deficiencies, and therefore presumably treatable by the administration of evening primrose oil, are exceedingly numerous. The more significant ones in terms of supporting evidence are PMS and associated mastalgia, as well as atopic eczema. However, even in these conditions, which have been the subject of a number of studies, the results are controversial.

A comprehensive literature review, published in 1989, reported that evening primrose had some utility in treating PMS,[16] but a 1990 clinical study concluded that the improvement was solely a placebo effect.[17] The same criticism has been leveled against the use of the oil in treating atopic eczema.[18] In view of this uncertainty regarding the efficacy of evening primrose oil and the relatively high cost of the 500 mg. capsules (ca. $.25 ea–minimum dose, 4 per day), it is not possible to endorse the use of this product. This position is further supported by the lack of toxicity data regarding long-term use of the product.

In 1992, the Food and Drug Administration took the position that evening primrose oil was an unapproved food additive and not generally recognized as safe for human consumption. This conclusion, upheld by federal court decisions, led to the seizure of wholesale stocks of the product.[19]

GLA-rich seed oils from two other plant sources are currently available in the United States.

Black Currant Oil

The seed of *Ribes nigrum* L., family Grossulariaceae, the European black currant, yields a fixed oil containing 14 to 19 percent GLA. Capsules containing approximately 200 or 400 mg. of the product are currently marketed.

Borage Seed Oil

Obtained from the seed of *Borago officinalis* L., family Boraginaceae, this oil contains 20 to 26 percent of GLA.[15] It is presently marketed in the form of capsules, each containing 1,300 mg. of the oil equivalent to 300 mg. of GLA. Borage seeds have been shown to contain small amounts of pyrrolizidine alkaloids, including the known hepatotoxin amabiline. That alkaloid was not detected in samples of the seed oil down to levels of 5 μg./g. Consumption of 1 to 2 g. of borage seed oil daily could, nevertheless, result in an intake of toxic unsaturated pyrrolizidine alkaloids (UPAs) approaching 10 μg. As De Smet has pointed out, the German Federal Health Agency now limits internal consumption of such products to not more than 1 μg. of UPA daily.[20] This means that in the interest of consumer safety, borage seed oil should be certified free of UPAs down to the level of 0.5 to 1 μg./g.

The fact that GLA-rich fatty oils are now available commercially from three different plant sources does not alter the conclusion that the product's efficacy for any condition remains unproven. Likewise, its safety on long-term usage requires additional verification. This is especially important for borage seed oil, which may contain small amounts of UPAs.

Raspberry Leaves

Raspberry leaf tea, an infusion prepared from the dried leaves of *Rubus idaeus* L. or *R. strigosus* Michx. of the family Rosaceae, has a considerable reputation as "a traditional remedy for painful and profuse menstruation and for use before and during confinement to make partruition easier and speedier."[21] Because of its astringent properties, it is also used to treat diarrhea, an application previously discussed in Chapter 4. The scientific evidence supporting the effects of raspberry leaves on the uterus is scanty, and clinical evidence is nonexistent.

Beckett and colleagues carried out the most substantial pharmacological testing to date, using isolated tissues of guinea pigs and frogs.[22] They concluded that aqueous raspberry leaf extracts contain a number of different active constituents, the actions of which are mutually antagonistic. These include: (1) a smooth muscle stimulant, (2) an anticholinesterase, and (3) a spasmolytic. They noted that it would be impossible to predict an overall clinical effect.

There is also a difference in the effect of the herb on pregnant versus non-pregnant human uterine strips. It was without effect on the latter but promoted contraction of normal human uterine strips at 10 to 16 weeks of pregnancy.[23] Such findings seriously complicate any attempt at the evaluation of the efficacy of the herb for any of its folkloric uses. Evaluation is further hampered by the absence of any long-term toxicity data, including teratogenicity. This is an especially serious omission in view of the fact that one of the recommended uses of raspberry leaf tea is to alleviate morning sickness.[24] Doses also are relatively large. At least one source recommends preparing a tea by steeping 30 g. (1 oz.) of leaves in 480 ml. (1 pint) of boiling water for 30 minutes and drinking the entire quantity to promote an easy labor.[25] A more reasonable dose is prepared by steeping about 2 g. (1 teaspoonful) of the leaves in 240 ml. (1 cup) of boiling water for 5 minutes.

In view of these factors, it seems best to adhere to the admonition that the consumption of any herbal product of unproven safety and efficacy is especially unwise during pregnancy. Deviation from this rule will certainly produce more harm than good.

HYPERTHYROIDISM

Also referred to as thyrotoxicosis or Graves' disease, hyperthyroidism is a very common endocrine disorder that may arise from a number of different causes. It is characterized by symptoms that may include weakness, weight loss, nervousness, tachycardia, exophthalmos, and goiter.

Bugle Weed

An herb that has been used to treat the condition is bugle weed. It consists of the leaves and tops collected before flowering of *Lycopus virginicus* L. or *L. europaeus* L. of the family Lamiaceae. The principles responsible for bugle weed's antithyrotropic function have not been identified.[5] Hyperthyroidism is a complex disease scarcely amenable to self-treatment with nonstandardized medicaments. Consequently, bugle weed will not be further considered here.

DIABETES MELLITUS

This condition is characterized by inappropriate hyperglycemia resulting either from a deficiency of insulin, or a reduction in its effectiveness, or both. The condition is normally treated either by diet, by the administration of exogenous insulin, or by the use of oral hypoglycemic drugs. These latter function, at least in part, by stimulating the beta cells of the pancreas to produce more insulin.

A large number of plants have been shown to exert hypoglycemic effects in small animal studies. None of these plants has been adequately tested in human beings to demonstrate conclusively its safety and utility as a substitute either for insulin or for the oral hypoglycemic drugs.[26] Further, none of them is currently marketed in the form of a preparation with standardized activity. This would be an absolute necessity if it were to be used to control hyperglycemia successfully. For these reasons, none of the so-called antidiabetic herbs will be discussed here.

REFERENCE NOTES

1. Strobl, J. and Thomas, J.A.: "Chapter 66" in *Modern Pharmacology*, 3rd ed., C.R. Craig and R.E. Stitzel, eds., Little, Brown, Boston, 1990, pp. 882-884.

2. Keye, W.R., Jr.: "Premenstrual Syndrome (PMS)" in *Conn's Current Therapy*, H.F. Conn and R.E. Rakel, eds., W.B. Saunders, Philadelphia, 1984, pp. 1000-1003.

3. Nelson, R.: "Dysmenorrhea" in *Conn's Current Therapy*, H.F. Conn and R.E. Rakel, eds. W.B. Saunders, Philadelphia, 1984 pp. 999-1000.

4. Burton, J.: *Lydia Pinkham Is Her Name*, Farrar, Straus, New York, 1949, p. 107.

5. Hänsel, R.: *Phytopharmaka*, 2nd ed., Springer-Verlag, Berlin, 1991, pp. 223-230.

6. Lehmann-Willenbrock, E. and Riedel, H.H.: *Zentralblatt für Gynäkologie* **110**:611-618 (1988).

7. Düker, E.-M., Kopanski, L., Jarry, H., and Wuttke, W.: *Planta Medica* **57**:420-424 (1991).

8. *Bundesanzeiger* (Cologne, Germany): January 5, 1989.

9. Blumenthal, M.: *Health Foods Business* **35**(9):18, 104-105 (1989).

10. Winterhoff, H., Gorkow, C., and Behr, B.: *Zeitschrift für Phytotherapie* **12**:175-179 (1991).

11. Thomas, J.A.: "Chapter 63" in *Modern Pharmacology,* 3rd ed., C.R. Craig and R.E. Stitzel, eds., Little, Brown, Boston, 1990, p. 850.

12. *Bundesanzeiger* (Cologne, Germany): May 15, 1985.

13. Briggs, C.J.: *Canadian Pharmaceutical Journal* **119**:248-254 (1986).

14. Barber, A.J.: *Pharmaceutical Journal* **240**:723-725 (1988).

15. Awang, D.V.C.: *Canadian Pharmaceutical Journal* **123**:121-126 (1990).

16. *Lawrence Review of Natural Products:* March, 1989.

17. Khoo, S. K., Munro, C., and Battistutta, D.: *Medical Journal of Australia* **153**:189-192 (1990).

18. Sharpe, G.R. and Farr, P.M.: *Lancet* **335**:1283 (1990).

19. Anon.: *Health Foods Business* **38**(8):13 (1992).

20. De Smet, P.A.G.M. : *Canadian Pharmaceutical Journal* **124**:5 (1991).

21. *The Extra Pharmacopoeia–Martindale,* 24th ed., vol. 1, The Pharmaceutical Press, London, 1958, p. 614.

22. Beckett, A.H., Belthle, F.W., Fell, K.R., and Lockett, M.F.: *Journal of Pharmacy and Pharmacology* **6**:785-796 (1954).

23. Bamford, D.S., Percival, R.C., and Tothill, A.U.: *British Journal of Pharmacology* **40**:161P-162P (1970).

24. Castleman, M.: *The Healing Herbs,* Rodale Press, Emmaus, Pennsylvania, 1991, pp. 294-296.

25. Bricklin, M.: *Encyclopedia of Natural Home Remedies,* Rodale Press, Emmaus, Pennsylvania, 1982, pp. 379-381.

26. Weiss, R. F.: *Herbal Medicine,* AB Arcanum, Gothenburg, Sweden, 1988, pp. 275-278.

Chapter 10

Arthritic and Musculoskeletal Disorders

ARTHRITIS

Arthritis refers to a whole spectrum of disorders, all of which are characterized by inflammation and tissue damage at the joints. Some of the various types are rheumatoid arthritis, juvenile arthritis, ankylosing spondylitis, psoriatic arthritis, Reiter's syndrome, osteoarthritis, and fibrositic disorders. Of these, rheumatoid arthritis is the most common, occurring in about 1 percent of the adult population and 2 to 3 times more often in women than in men. Its cause is thought by many to be an infection, yet years of searching have not revealed a causative organism. Regardless of the type of arthritis, the immune response plays a significant role in producing both local inflammation and tissue damage.[1]

Initial drug therapy of most of the types of arthritis involves the systemic administration of salicylates. Administered in sufficient doses, these compounds reduce inflammation, provide a degree of analgesia, maintain joint mobility, and help prevent deformity. They do not, however, alter the long-term progression of the disease.[2] While aspirin is the salicylate of choice for treating arthritis, some persons advocate the use of the herb:

Willow Bark

About 300 different species of the genus *Salix* are called willow. The one that is generally recognized as a source of medicinal bark in the United States is *Salix alba* L., but for reasons that will become clear, the bark of *Salix purpurea* L. and *Salix fragilis* L. are of superior quality.

The principal active constituent of willow bark was long thought to be a compound known as salicin, which chemically is salicyl alcohol glycoside. However, recent studies have shown that a whole series of phenolic glycosides designated salicortin (normally the main active principle in willow species), fragilin, tremulacin, etc., are present in the bark, some in much larger amounts than true salicin.[3] The glycosides, other than salicin, are relatively heat labile and are converted to the latter compound if the bark is dried at a high temperature.[4] All of the phenolic glycosides have similar physiological effects, being pro-drugs that are converted to the active principle, salicylic acid, in the intestinal tract and the liver.[5] Because of the time required for this conversion, the therapeutic properties of willow bark are expressed more slowly but continue to be effective for a longer time than if salicylate itself were administered.[6]

For analytical purposes, the numerous phenolic glycosides are first converted to salicin and their content then indicated as total salicin per unit weight of dried bark. Such studies show an enormous variability, not only among different species of willow bark but also among different collections of the same species. Barks of high quality, such as those of *S. purpurea*, range from about 6 to 8.5 percent total salicin; one sample of *S. fragilis* even exceeded 10 percent. Probably a figure of 7 percent for such quality barks is about average. However, none of the *S. alba* samples exceeded 1 percent, and other willow species had even less. In Germany, a standard of not less than 1 percent total salicin has been established for willow bark. This is indicative of the low level of total salicin in most commercial samples.

Most of the willow bark available commercially is in the form of rather coarse pieces. Studies have shown that normal preparation of a tea from such material using hot water would extract only about 75 percent of the active principles. If a very finely powdered bark is used, the extraction will approach 100 percent of the activity.

The usual daily dose of aspirin for arthritic disorders is 3.6 to 5.4 g. (average 4.5 g.) administered in divided doses. Equivalent amounts of other salicylates are also effective. The question then becomes, how much total-salicin-containing willow bark must be administered to produce that amount of salicylate in the body? For purposes of this example, let us assume use of a relatively good quality bark containing 7 percent total salicin. Let us also assume that the bark is finely powdered and is carefully extracted with sufficient hot water to obtain 100 percent of the active principles. Because the exact composition of the mixture of phenolic glycosides (salicin, salicortin, etc.) varies in the individual barks, it is not possible to calculate the exact amount of active salicylate produced from a given quantity of an unknown mixture. Theoretically, it will be considerably less than 50 percent, and that conversion will occur over several hours, not immediately. But for convenience in calculating, let us assume 50 percent.

Based on these generous assumptions, it would be necessary to consume the tea prepared from about 130 g. of bark to yield an average daily dose of salicylate sufficient to treat arthritic-rheumatic disorders. In the calculations that follow, figures have been rounded off and should be viewed as approximations. At the standard strength of 1 teaspoonful (1.5 g.) per cup (240 ml.) of water, that is more than 20 liters (5 1/2 gallons) of willow tea daily. Considering the high concentration of tannin (8-20 percent) in the bark and the sheer volume of liquid involved, consumption of this quantity is not physically possible. If ordinary willow bark with its approximately 1 percent total salicin were to be substituted for the superior quality bark, these figures must be multiplied by 7, yielding 2 pounds (1 kg.) of bark and some 38 gallons (140 liters) of tea–an utterly impossible daily dose. The need for such high dosage levels also precludes effective use of the crude herb in another form such as capsules or tablets.

What about the use of willow bark for other conditions–headache, fever, sprains, strains, etc.–that respond to treatment with salicylates? Here, there is liable to be confusion about proper dosage because the German Commission E recommends use of a quantity of bark equivalent to 60 to 120 mg. of total salicin daily. Such a minimal dose would have little therapeutic value and seems to be based more on the quantity of bark used to prepare a normal cup of tea than upon any proven value of the small amount of total salicin contained therein. It does also point out that willow bark is used in German medicine as an adjuvant or auxiliary drug, not as an agent which, in itself, possesses great therapeutic value. In practice, it is supplemented by administration of synthetic salicylates.[6,7]

The National Formulary VI listed the average dose of salicin as 1 g.[8] This is a reasonable analgesic-antipyretic dose, considering that the compound has less than one-half the activity of salicylates. It would require approximately 14 g. (1/2 ounce or 10 heaping tea-spoonfuls) of high quality willow bark (7 percent total salicin) prepared as 10 cups (240 ml. ea.) of tea to yield a single average dose of salicin. If ordinary white willow bark were employed, these quantities would have to be multiplied by 7.

In spite of the presence in various willow barks of total salicin, a mixture of therapeutically/useful salicylate precursors, these herbs by themselves do not constitute effective treatment for arthritis or even for headaches, fevers, or muscle pains. The quantity of active principles present in even the highest quality barks is insufficient to allow them to be consumed in sufficient amounts to constitute useful medicines. They may play a psychologically supportive role as auxiliaries to synthetic salicylate therapy in certain patients.

MUSCLE PAIN

External analgesics, many of which are of plant origin, are widely used to allay the discomfort associated with the overuse of skeletal muscles. When stimulated by strenuous exercise or other irritations, pain receptors located in the skeletal muscles transmit impulses to the brain, which are interpreted as pain. Such deep-seated pain is difficult to characterize; it is often described as "dull" or "aching."[9]

Pain of this sort is often treated with an external analgesic that functions as a counterirritant; that is, it provides a mild local inflammatory reaction over or near the site of the underlying pain. Many counterirritants are also rubefacients, producing dilation of the cutaneous vasculature and subsequent reddening of the skin. The resulting localized reaction of warmth and redness causes the patient to disregard the original deep-seated pain. Many theories have been proposed to explain the functioning of counterirritants, but none is completely satisfactory. Probably the pain-relieving effect has a strong placebo component.[10]

Rubefacients (Agents that Induce Redness and Irritation)

Volatile Mustard Oil (Allyl Isothiocyanate)

This is a volatile oil obtained from the dried ripe seed of varieties of black mustard, *Brassica nigra* (L.) W.D.J. Koch or of *B. juncea* (L.) Czern. var. *timida* Tsen & Lee, family Brassicaceae.[11] The seed is ground, then macerated in water to allow the enzyme myrosin to convert the glycoside sinigrin to allyl isothiocyanate. This volatile compound is then purified by distillation and incorporated into various counterirritant preparations intended for external application.

Alternatively, a poultice may be prepared from equal parts of the powdered seeds and flour by moistening with sufficient water to form a paste. The mixture is spread on a cloth and applied to the affected area for a short period of time. If left too long, the continued release of the volatile mustard oil may blister the skin.

Although it is extremely acrid and irritating, volatile mustard oil is considered by the FDA to be a safe and effective counterirritant if applied in concentrations ranging from 0.5 to 5.0 percent. It may be used as frequently as 3 or 4 times daily.

Methyl Salicylate

This compound is obtained by distilling the leaves of wintergreen, *Gaultheria procumbens* L. (family Ericaceae) or the bark of the sweet birch, *Betula lenta* L. (family Betulaceae). These products are referred to as wintergreen oil and sweet birch oil, respectively. They are essentially indistinguishable from each other and from methyl salicylate that is prepared synthetically by the esterification of synthetic salicylic acid.[12]

Methyl salicylate is applied topically as a counterirritant in the form of liniments, gels, lotions, or ointments containing concentrations of 10 to 60 percent. The number of applications should not exceed 3 or 4 per day. Strenuous physical activity and heat increase

the percutaneous absorption of methyl salicylate, which may result
in salicylate toxicity. Consequently, users should be warned not to
apply methyl salicylate after vigorous exercise in hot and humid
weather or to follow up the application by use of a heating pad.[10]

Turpentine Oil

Sometimes called Spirits of Turpentine, this is a volatile oil distilled from the oleoresin obtained from the long-leaf pine, *Pinus
palustris* Mill., family Pinaceae. It has a long history of use in
counterirritant preparations, being employed in concentrations of 6
to 50 percent. Application should not exceed 3 or 4 times daily.

Refrigerants (Agents that Induce a Cooling Sensation)

There are two additional products that are slightly less effective
than those counterirritants previously discussed but which are nevertheless widely used. Both differ from the previous ones in that
they produce a strong cooling sensation when applied to the skin.

Menthol

This is an alcohol obtained from various mint oils or produced
synthetically. It is employed 3 or 4 times a day in topical preparations in concentrations of 0.1 to 1.0 percent.

Camphor

Camphor is a ketone obtained from *Cinnamomum camphora* (L.)
J.S. Presl of the family Lauraceae, or produced synthetically. It is
used 3 or 4 times daily as a counterirritant in topical preparations
containing concentrations of 0.1 to 3.0 percent.

Other Counterirritants

The **Capsicum**-derived capsaicin cream discussed in Chapter 8
as a pain controller also provides counterirritant activity but without
rubefaction. For details of its composition and use, see the discussion there.

GOUT

Gout is a recurrent form of acute arthritis resulting from a deposition of crystals of monosodium urate in and around the joints and tendons. It is extremely painful, and if not treated, can lead to chronic disability.[13]

Colchicum

One of the most ancient treatments for gout is Colchicum. For more than 500 years the corm of the autumn crocus, *Colchicum autumnale* L. of the family Liliaceae, has been used as a specific treatment to alleviate the inflammation associated with gout. Then, about 150 years ago, colchicum seeds began to be utilized for the same purpose. In 1820, the active principle colchicine was first isolated, and in the intervening years, it has replaced the herb (corm and seed) as the dosage form of choice. In therapeutic doses, colchicine displays a number of unpleasant side effects, and in large doses, it is quite toxic.[14] As a result, neither it nor the plant material containing it is available for over-the-counter acquisition. It will not be discussed further here.

REFERENCE NOTES

1. *Drug Evaluations*, 6th ed., American Medical Association, 1986, p. 1049.

2. Kvam, D.C. and Swingle, K.F.: "Chapter 43" in *Modern Pharmacology*, 3rd ed., C.R. Craig and R.E. Stitzel, eds., Little, Brown, Boston, 1990, pp. 570-590.

3. Meier, B., Sticher, O., and Bettschart, A.: *Deutsche Apotheker Zeitung* **125**:341-347 (1985).

4. Julkunen-Tiitto, R. and Gebhardt, K.: *Planta Medica* **58**:385-386 (1992).

5. Meier, B. and Liebi, M.: *Zeitschrift für Phytotherapie* **11**:50-58 (1990).

6. Schneider, E.: *Zeitschrift für Phytotherapie* 8:35-37 (1987).

7. Hänsel, R. and Haas, H.: *Therapie mit Phytopharmaka*, Springer-Verlag, Berlin, 1984, pp. 233-235.

8. *The National Formulary*, 6th ed., American Pharmaceutical Association, Washington, D.C., 1935, pp. 322-323.

9 Gossel, T.A.: *U.S. Pharmacist* **12**(8):26-36, 105 (1987).

10. Jacknowitz, A.I.: "Chapter 32" in *Handbook of Nonprescription Drugs*, 9th ed., American Pharmaceutical Association, Washington, D.C., 1990, pp. 872-883.

11. Tyler, V.E., Brady, L.R., and Robbers, J.E.: *Pharmacognosy*, 9th ed., Lea & Febiger, Philadelphia, 1988, pp. 72-73.

12. Osol, A. and Farrar, G.E., Jr.: *The Dispensatory of the United States of America*, 24th ed., J. B. Lippincott, Philadelphia, 1947, pp. 707-708.

13. *Professional Guide to Diseases*, 3rd ed., Springhouse, Springhouse, Pennsylvania, 1989, p. 525.

14. Van Dyke, K.: "Chapter 44" in *Modern Pharmacology*, 3rd ed., C.R. Craig and R.E. Stitzel, eds., Little, Brown, Boston, 1990, pp. 591-600.

Chapter 11

Problems of the Skin, Mucous Membranes, and Gingiva

DERMATITIS

Dermatitis is not so much a disease as it is a symptom, an erythematous condition of the skin characterized by inflammation and redness. It may result from various external or internal causative factors. The condition is typified by pruritis or itching and initial weeping of the skin, giving way in time to a dry, scaly condition.

Herbal treatment of dermatitis is a conservative therapy involving, first of all, removal of the irritating or allergenic agent from the environment. Soaps and detergents are primary causative agents if the hands are involved. This is followed by application of a solution with astringent properties to reduce the weeping. Such solutions generally function by coagulating the surface proteins of the cells, reducing their permeability, and limiting the secretion of the inflamed tissue. The precipitated proteins also tend to form a protective layer, thereby limiting bacterial development and facilitating the growth underneath of new tissue. Tannin-containing herbs are especially effective astringents.[1]

Tannin-Containing Herbs

Witch Hazel Leaves

One of the most widely used herbs in this category is witch hazel leaves. Also known as hamamelis leaves, this herb consists of the dried leaves of *Hamamelis virginiana* L., a native American shrub or small tree of the family Hamamelidaceae. The leaves contain 8 to 10 percent of a mixture of tannins, consisting chiefly of gallotannins with some condensed catechins and proanthocyanins.[2] An aqueous or hydroalcoholic extract of witch hazel leaves contains large amounts of tannin and is an excellent astringent. Unfortunately, such preparations are not ordinarily available in the United States. The only common commercial product here is technically referred to as hamamelis water, witch hazel extract, or distilled witch hazel extract; however, in the vernacular it is known simply as witch hazel.

Distilled witch hazel extract is prepared by macerating in water and then steam distilling the recently cut, dormant twigs of the plant. Alcohol is then added to the distillate to obtain a final concentration of 14 to 15 percent. It is this product, prepared according to the procedure described in the *NF XI* in 1960, that the FDA has declared, under the colloquial designation "witch hazel," to be a safe and effective astringent. Since the tannins are not carried over into the extract during the distillation process, the only plant constituent present is a trace of volatile oil too limited in amount to exert any therapeutic influence. Whatever astringent activity is present, and that must be very limited indeed, can be attributed only to the 14 to 15 percent alcohol contained in the product.

Authentic (nondistilled) hydroalcoholic extracts of witch hazel leaves are, on the other hand, much more effective astringents and styptics. They are used, either as such or following incorporation into an ointment base, to relieve local inflammation of the skin and mucous membranes.

Oak Bark

When this product was an official drug in the *NF*, it was said to consist of the dried inner bark of the trunk and branches of the white oak, *Quercus alba* L. of the family Fagaceae. However, the barks of a number of different oaks have been used medicinally, including *Q. robur* L., the British oak, and *Q. petraea* (Matt.) Liebl., the winter oak. Oak bark contains 6 to 11 percent of a characteristic tannin known as quercitannic acid.[3] For local use, a decoction is prepared from 2 teaspoonfuls (6 g.) of the coarsely powdered bark and 500 ml. (1 pint) of water. After straining, this aqueous extract is applied directly to the affected skin; it is also used as a mouthwash for inflammation of the mucous membranes of the oral cavity.[4]

English Walnut Leaves

The dried leaves of the English walnut, *Juglans regia* L., family Juglandaceae, contain about 10 percent of an ellagic acid-derived tannin and are therefore utilized as a local astringent in a manner similar to the preceding herbs. A decoction prepared by boiling 5 teaspoonfuls (5 g.) of the leaves in 200 ml. (ca. 1 cup) of water, then straining, is applied to the affected skin 3 or 4 times a day.[5]

Other Herbal Products

As noted previously, a number of ointments, creams, and lotions containing **Chamomile Volatile Oil** and intended for the treatment of various skin conditions are currently marketed in Europe. Since these pharmaceuticals have not been approved for sale in the United States, and consequently are not available here, they are not discussed in this chapter. See Chapter 4 for a detailed discussion of this herb.

Evening Primrose Oil, previously discussed, has been thought to be of value in treating atopic eczema (dermatitis). However, conclusive proof of its value in such conditions is lacking.

CONTACT DERMATITIS

The most severe type of acute contact dermatitis is that produced by touching poison ivy, *Toxicodendron radicans* (L.) O. Kuntze or other related species of *Toxicondendron* known as poison oak or poison sumac. A toxic mixture of catechols designated urushiol is contained in this species. Following initial sensitization, it produces an acute contact dermatitis characterized by weeping, vesicular lesions with edema, crusting, and occasionally secondary infection. Itching may be severe. Conventional treatment, depending on the severity of the condition, involves the systemic or local administration of corticosteroids and drying lotions applied to the lesions.[6]

More than 100 different plants or plant products have been used in the past to treat poison ivy.

Jewelweed

The most effective of these is probably jewelweed. In a study of Indiana folk medicine, the use of jewelweed, *Impatiens biflora* Walt. or *I. pallida* Nutt. (family Balsaminaceae), taken internally or applied externally, was repeatedly recommended as a cure for poison ivy dermatitis. Internally, a decoction prepared from any part of the plant is used; externally, the sap of the stem is applied to the affected area.[7]

The results of a clinical study, in which a 1:4 jewelweed preparation was compared for its effectiveness with other standard poison ivy dermatitis treatments were published in 1958.[8] Of the 115 patients treated with jewelweed, 108 responded "most dramatically to the topical application of this medication and were entirely relieved of their symptoms within 2 or 3 days after the institution of treatment." It was concluded that jewelweed is an excellent substitute for ACTH and the corticosteroids in the treatment of poison ivy dermatitis. The active principle in the plant responsible for this activity remains unidentified.

BURNS, WOUNDS, AND INFECTIONS

Because a single herbal remedy is often used to treat two or more of these conditions, they are all considered in a single section. Burns and wounds require treatment to alleviate pain, to prevent infection, and to facilitate regeneration of tissue. Both occur quite commonly, especially in the home. For example, 80 percent of the burns occur there, but only 5 percent are severe enough to require hospitalization. Of the minor burns occurring outside the home, sunburn is the most common. The goals of treating minor burns (those not affecting full-skin thickness) are to relieve the pain, protect it from air, prevent dryness, and provide a favorable environment for healing without infection.[9]

Abrasions or minor cuts or wounds are normally cleansed to remove debris that might lead to infection, and an antiseptic preparation is applied. Ideally, such an antiseptic should be minimally affected by the presence of organic materials. Such preparations often stain the tissue. While this is generally undesirable, it may be useful in delineating a "clean" area.[10]

A relatively large number of fungal infections of the skin occur in human beings. These include ringworm of the scalp or body, jock itch, athlete's foot, candidiasis, and the like.[11] Normally, such conditions are treated by the topical application of antifungal agents, although in stubborn cases it may be necessary to resort to the systemic administration of appropriate antibiotics.

In recent years, the incidence of so-called vaginal yeast infections has increased somewhat, but public awareness of the condition has increased markedly. The common causative agent is not a true yeast but rather *Candida albicans* (or a related *Candida* species), an imperfect fungus with a yeast-like appearance. The increased incidence is attributed to more widespread use of broad spectrum antibiotics, which permit candida infections to develop by destroying the normal vaginal flora, and to the popularity of occlusive female clothing, particularly panty hose. Public awareness has been promoted by extensive advertising of two synthetic vaginal fungicides, clotrimazole and miconazole, that were switched to OTC status in 1991.

Aloe

One of the most widely used herbal preparations for the treatment of various skin conditions is aloe. Often referred to as aloe vera or aloe gel, this is the mucilaginous gel obtained from the cells making up the inner portion (parenchyma) of the leaf of *Aloë barbadensis* Mill. (family Liliaceae), sometimes referred to as *A. vera* (L.) N. L. Burm. or *A. vulgaris* Lam. The gel should not be confused with the bitter yellow latex or juice that derives from the pericyclic tubules occurring just beneath the epidermis or rind of the leaves. That material, in dried form, is a potent laxative and has been previously discussed in Chapter 4.[12]

Aloe gel has been widely used externally for its wound healing properties and internally as a general tonic or cure-all. It is incorporated into a wide variety of ointments, creams, lotions, shampoos, and the like for external use. While there appears to be general agreement regarding the effectiveness of fresh aloe gel in the treatment of minor skin ailments, there is considerable controversy on the effectiveness of these aloe preparations. In the first place, the gel is often obtained and treated in different ways. Some of it is even "reconstituted" from a powder or concentrated liquid. "Aloe vera extract" usually denotes a diluted product.[13] These differences in processing and the resulting composition of the product have resulted in differences in observed activity of the commercial products.

One study of the effect of aloe gel on the growth of human cells in artificial culture found that the fresh material significantly promoted the attachment and growth of the cells. It also enhanced the healing of wounded monolayers of the cells. However, a "stabilized" commercial product actually proved toxic to such cells, disrupting their attachment and growth.[14] A subsequent study of 21 patients with wound complications following cesarean section or laparotomy showed that treatment with a commercial aloe gel preparation (production method unspecified) significantly delayed wound healing.[15]

Other studies, however, have shown that aloe gel and some preparations containing it were useful in the treatment of various types of skin ulceration in humans, and burn and frostbite injuries in animals.[16] In another study, a cream base containing aloe was shown to be effective in preserving circulation in the skin after frostbite injury.[17] Stabilized aloe vera was shown to produce a dramatic acceleration of wound healing in patients who had undergone full-face dermabrasion.[18] Thus, evidence is beginning to accumulate to support not only the effectiveness of fresh aloe gel but also some preparations containing the processed product.

It is presently believed that some of the beneficial effects of aloe apparently result from the ability of a contained carboxypeptidase to inhibit the pain-producing agent bradykinin. The product is also believed to hinder the formation of thromboxane, the activity of which is detrimental to burn wound healing. Antiprostaglandin activity has also been reported. Aloe gel has antibacterial and antifungal properties, but little is known about the identity and stability of the ingredients responsible for these or most of its other effects. Many of the active constituents undoubtedly deteriorate on storage, so use of the fresh gel is the only way to assure maximal activity. Although the FDA concluded that there was insufficient evidence to support the effectiveness of aloe gel in treating any condition,[19] the product continues to be widely used as a remedy for minor skin ailments–cuts, bruises, abrasions, burns, etc.

Arnica

The dried flower heads of *Arnica montana* L. (family Asteraceae) and several other related species of *Arnica* have a longstanding reputation as a useful treatment for acne, bruises, sprains, muscle aches, and as a general topical counterirritant. The plant contains a number of sesquiterpene lactones, flavonoid glycosides, and about 1 percent of a volatile oil.[20] Two isomeric alcohols, arnidiol and foradiol, have been shown to act as counterirritants. In animal experiments, the sesquiterpene lactone helenalin reduces the inflammatory process and the formation of edema.[21] Unfortunately, helenalin and its derivatives are also allergenic and may induce topical dermatitis.[22]

In this country, arnica is commonly employed in the form of a tincture (hydroalcoholic extract) that is applied externally to the area to be treated. In Europe, arnica-containing creams are especially popular. The herb is approved by German Commission E for its anti-inflammatory, analgesic, and antiseptic properties on topical application.[23] It should not be taken internally.

Calendula

The ligulate florets, often erroneously called petals, of *Calendula officinalis* L. (family Asteraceae), commonly known as the garden marigold, have long been valued in Europe for the treatment of various skin ailments and to facilitate wound healing. Chemical principles responsible for these effects remain unidentified.[24]

Calendula is utilized in the form of a tea prepared by pouring 1 cup (240 ml.) of boiling water over 1 to 2 teaspoonfuls (1-1.5 g.) of herb and allowing it to steep for 10 minutes. This preparation is used as a gargle or mouthwash for sores in the mouth or poured over an absorbent cloth and applied as a poultice to skin ailments. Occasionally, the tea is even consumed internally for its antispasmodic and other putative effects.[25] Extract of calendula is also incorporated into soaps as well as various ointments, creams, and sprays intended for local application. German Commission E has found calendula to be effective for the reduction of inflammation and promotion of granulation of wounds.[26] In short, it promotes wound healing on local application.

Comfrey

This herb, also called common comfrey, should consist of the leaves or the root of *Symphytum officinale* L. of the family Boraginaceae; however, in commercial practice today it is seldom differentiated from prickly comfrey, *S. asperum* Lepech., or from Russian comfrey, *S.* x *uplandicum* Nym. Comfrey was initially applied externally to reduce the swelling around broken bones. Then it began to be used for treating a variety of wounds and, more recently, internally as a kind of tonic.[27]

Whatever therapeutic value comfrey may possess is attributed to its content of allantoin, a cell proliferant, and to rosmarinic acid, an anti-inflammatory agent and inhibitor of microvascular pulmonary injury.[28,29] Unfortunately, these beneficial principles are accompanied in the herb by a large number of toxic pyrrolizidine alkaloids that have been shown to cause cancer in small animals. Four cases of human poisoning by comfrey have now been reported, although it is not certain if all of them resulted from the ingestion of *S. officinale* (common comfrey). The identity of the species is important because it is now recognized that, although *S. officinale* contains toxic pyrrolizidine alkaloids (PAs), it usually does not contain large quantities of the extremely dangerous echimidine found in *S. asperum* (prickly comfrey) or *S.* x *uplandicum* (Russian comfrey).[30] Originally, it was believed that *S. officinale* did not contain echimidine, but a 1989 chemotaxonomic study revealed that about one-fourth of the common comfrey samples examined did contain that alkaloid, although generally in very small amounts.[31] It is still reasonable to conclude that a high level of echimidine in a comfrey sample indicates a species other than *S. officinale*.

Awang[30] has shown that about half of the comfrey products available in Canada contained echimidine, in spite of the fact that they were labeled as consisting of common comfrey. This inattention to proper taxonomic identification by suppliers creates a particularly dangerous situation. In addition, comfrey roots contain about ten times the concentration of PAs found in leaves, rendering the roots unsuitable for any therapeutic application. Health and Welfare Canada has long refused to register any comfrey root products for medicinal application.

Reflecting its former enormous popularity, comfrey continues to be used both externally and internally by many people who are misinformed by advice provided in popular herbals. Believing that the use of herbs should be helpful, not harmful, to the consumers health, it must be concluded:

1. The internal use of any species of comfrey should be avoided.
2. Comfrey root should never be used medicinally.
3. Only the mature leaves of *S. officinale* should be applied externally, and then only to intact skin for limited periods of time.
4. Comfrey should never be used by pregnant or lactating women or by young children.
5. Because there are so many other nontoxic yet effective treatments for minor skin ailments that do not present the hazards associated with this herb, comfrey has little, if any, place in our modern materia medica.

In 1992, the German Federal Health Agency, in an attempt to balance the popularity of certain herbs containing toxic PAs with a recognized need for their restricted usage, established standards for such preparations. These limitations restricted the amount of total PAs with 1,2-unsaturated necine moieties that might be obtained from certain registered preparations to not more than 100 μg. per day when used externally and 1 μg. per day when taken internally. An exception was made for comfrey leaf tea, which was permitted to provide a maximum internal daily dose of 10 μg. In the case of non-registered preparations, the limitations were reduced to 10 μg. externally and 0.1 μg. internally daily.[32]

It is necessary to point out that these limitations, which apply not only to comfrey but to such other herbs as borage, coltsfoot, life root, and heliotrope, are meaningless in the United States because none of the preparations sold here has been assayed to determine its content of PAs. Further, no adjustment has been made in any of the available dosage forms to assure that these levels of toxic alkaloids are not exceeded. For this reason, safety requires adherence to the five rules stated above when dealing with comfrey. Similar precautions should be taken with all herbs containing toxic PAs.

Tea Tree Oil

When distilled with steam, the leaves of an Australian tree, *Melaleuca alternifolia* (Maiden & Betche) Cheel of the family Myrtaceae, yield about 2 percent of a pale yellow oil known as tea tree oil. About one-third of the oil is composed of terpene hydrocarbons (pinene, terpinene, cymene); the residual two-thirds consists primarily of oxygenated terpenes, particularly terpinen-4-ol, which may constitute up to 60 percent of the total oil. Sesquiterpene hydrocarbons and oxygenated sesquiterpenes are also present.[33]

The oil was said to have been used by the aborigines as a local antiseptic, and early settlers in Australia utilized it for the treatment of cuts, abrasions, burns, insect bites, athlete's foot, and the like.[34] Because of the presence of large amounts of terpinen-4-ol, the tea tree oil does possess a pronounced germicidal activity. In fact, during World War II, it was incorporated in the machine "cutting" oils used in munitions factories in Australia to reduce the number of infections resulting from the metal filings and turnings that accidentally penetrated the skin of the workers' hands.[35]

A very few modern clinical studies have shown the possible value of tea tree oil in treating various vaginal and skin infections and acne vulgaris.[36,37,38] Although irritation of the skin occasionally occurs in sensitive individuals, the use of the oil has not been associated with any particular toxicity. The oil is applied locally in concentrations ranging from 0.4 to 100 percent, depending on the nature and location of the condition requiring treatment.

Yogurt

This is a semisolid, curdled or coagulated milk product resulting from the action of certain bacteria on the sugars in milk. Classically, two organisms are used in combination, *Lactobacillus bulgaricus* and *Streptococcus thermophilus,* which are allowed to act on whole fresh cow's milk at a temperature of 40° to 50° C for a period of 5 to 10 hours.[39] In modern "low-fat" or "no-fat" yogurts, skim milk powder is added to milk with a reduced butterfat content to improve the consistency of the product, and the mixture is fermented with the above bacteria and/or *Lactobacillus acidophilus*. Although yogurt is certainly not an herb, it may be thought of in this case as simply a substrate for the bacteria that are traditionally classified as microscopic plants. Consequently, it is the therapeutic utility of the living plants that is really being discussed here.

Results of a clinical study published in 1992 showed that the daily consumption for a six-month period of 8 oz. (240 g.) of yogurt containing live *L. acidophilus* greatly reduced the incidence of recurrent candidal vaginitis.[40] Hilton and colleagues postulated that the bacteria colonized the gastrointestinal tract and then the vaginal canal where they restored or supplemented the normal lactobacilli flora and inhibited the growth of candida ("yeast").[40] As a result of these findings, the investigators recommended daily consumption of 1 cup (240 ml.) of yogurt containing live *L. acidophilus* bacteria to decrease both candidal colonization and infection of the vagina. The problem is that not all yogurts contain live cultures of this species. Further, the claims of dairy product manufacturers regarding the method of preparation of their various yogurts are not always accurate. Apparently, those most likely to contain *L. acidoph-ilus* are the low-fat, not the no-fat, varieties. Interested consumers can always make their own by following the directions provided for yogurt preparation in any reliable cookbook but using as a starter the contents of commercially available *L. acidophilus* capsules instead of a quantity of commercial yogurt. Alternatively, it seems reasonable to assume the consumption of the capsules themselves would produce the same results as the yogurt. Further clinical trials are definitely warranted.

LESIONS AND INFECTIONS
OF THE ORAL CAVITY AND THROAT

Various pain-inducing abnormalities of the oral cavity are quite common. Some 20 to 50 percent of Americans suffer from canker sores (recurrent aphthous ulcers), painful lesions apparently resulting from a dysfunction of the immune system. Virus-induced cold sores or fever blisters (herpes simplex) are also common as is stomatitis, an inflammation often associated with a systemic disease. Periodontal disease, such as gingivitis and Vincent's infection, are likewise seen with some frequency. Candidiasis, a fungal infection with *Candida*, is not uncommon.[41,42]

Canker Sores and Sore Throat

Although not necessarily related in origin, the same botanicals are used to treat both disorders, so it is convenient to consider them together here. Related ailments, such as cough, have already been discussed in Chapter 6. Many of these conditions are self-limiting; consequently, herbal treatments are, in general, palliative in character. Some of the commonly used herbs do possess modest antiseptic properties.

Goldenseal

Consisting of the dried rhizome and roots of *Hydrastis canadensis* L., family Ranunculaceae, this native American plant was introduced to the early settlers by the Cherokee Indians. It was long listed in the official compendia (*USP* and *NF*) and in relatively recent times was employed in medicine as a bitter. Previously, it had been thought to have value in treating urinary tract infections and in checking internal hemorrhage. However, there is no substantial clinical evidence that goldenseal or its constituents are effective in such conditions.[43]

Goldenseal contains a number of isoquinoline alkaloids, including hydrastine, berberine, and tetrahydroberberine. Of these, berberine is particularly active, having antibacterial and amoebicidal properties.[44] It probably accounts for the widespread use of goldenseal in the treatment of canker sores and other conditions causing sore mouth. A strong tea prepared from 2 teaspoonfuls (6 g.) of the herb and 1 cup (240 ml.) of water has a considerable folkloric reputation as a mouthwash to alleviate pain and facilitate healing. The process may be repeated 3 or 4 times daily. Lacking any modern clinical studies dealing with the safety and efficacy of goldenseal when used internally, it is necessary to agree with Sollmann that ingestion of the herb "has few, if any, rational indications."[43]

Rhatany

Containing more than 20 percent tannin, the dried root of *Krameria triandra* Ruiz & Pav., family Krameriaceae, is frequently used in the form of a hydroalcoholic solution (tincture) as a treatment for various oral lesions. Used either as such or combined with equal parts of myrrh tincture, it is applied locally to noninfectious canker sores with good results. Treatment is carried out 3 or 4 times daily. The tincture is also effective when used as a mouthwash, 1 or 2 teaspoonfuls (5-10 ml.) being added to a glass (300 ml.) of water for that purpose.[4]

Myrrh

Myrrh is neither a plant nor plant part; technically, it is an exudate, an oleo-gum-resin that exudes from incisions in the bark of *Commiphora molmol* Engl., *C. abyssinica* Engl., *C. myrrha* (Nees) Engl., or other species of the same genus (family Burseraceae). The plants yielding myrrh are small trees native to Ethiopia, Somalia, and the Arabian peninsula.[45] Consisting of a mixture of about 2.5 to 10 percent volatile oil, 50 to 60 percent gum, and 25 to 40 percent resin, the chemical constituents of myrrh are very complex. Presumably, its therapeutic utility may be attributed to the sesquiterpenes that dominate in the essential oil and to the resin acids in the resin. Many of the carbohydrate constituents comprising the gum are insoluble in alcohol and not found in the usual myrrh preparations.[46]

Utilized for many centuries for its astringent and protective properties, myrrh was first listed in the *USP* in 1820 and enjoyed official status there, and subsequently in the *NF*, until 1965. It is currently approved by the German Commission E for the local treatment of mild inflammations of the mucous membranes of the mouth and throat. Myrrh is almost always employed in the form of a tincture containing 20 percent of the drug in 85 percent alcohol. The tincture is applied locally to canker sores 2 or 3 times daily; a gargle for sore throat consists of 5 to 10 drops (0.25-0.5 ml.) of the tincture in a glass (300 ml.) of water.[47]

There are some preliminary indications that the oleo-gum-resin known variously as **Guggul** or **Guggulu** obtained from the related species *Commiphora mukul* Hook. may be effective in lowering blood cholesterol and triglyceride levels. Although guggul-based products containing so-called gugulipid are already marketed as drugs in India and France, and the powdered resin is available in the form of capsules in the United States, there is insufficient evidence available at this time to render a definitive judgment as to their safety and efficacy.[48] While preliminary indications are promising, much additional research is required to substantiate the value of the herb. Guggul was, therefore, not discussed in Chapter 7, "Cardiovascular System Problems." It is mentioned here merely to avoid confusing it with myrrh since both are derived from plants of the same genus.

Sage

The fresh or dried leaves of *Salvia officinalis* L. of the family Lamiaceae have a considerable reputation as a folkloric medicine. One herbal lists more than 60 different conditions for which the plant is said to be useful,[49] but most of the recommendations have not been validated scientifically. Sage leaves contain up to about 2.5 percent of a distinctive-smelling volatile oil in which thujone, the principal constituent (35-60 percent), is accompanied by cineole and other mono- and sesquiterpenes. About 3 to 7 percent of tannin is also present, as are bitter principles of the diterpene type.[50]

An infusion of sage prepared from 2 teaspoonfuls (3 g.) of finely cut plant material and a cup (240 ml.) of boiling water is widely used as a mouthwash or gargle for the treatment of inflammation of the mouth and throat. The volatile oil functions as an antiseptic, tannin as a local anti-inflammatory agent, and the bitter principles produce a pleasant sensory feeling in the mouth and throat.[51] The German Commission E has approved the external use of sage for these purposes, but it also allows its use internally for indigestion and to reduce excessive perspiration.[52] Although the herb may be effective in both conditions, the high thujone content of its volatile oil renders questionable the safety of frequent internal use. Both Wichtl and Commission E caution against overusage; in view of the high thujone content of sage oil, it seems wiser to restrict employment of sage preparations to use as mouthwashes or gargles.

Cold Sores

Often referred to as fever blisters, cold sores result from an infection with the herpes simplex type 1 virus. This condition is sometimes called herpes simplex labialis because the lesions usually develop on or around the lips where they tend to recur. Although they are both painful and unsightly, treatment is largely symptomatic, utilizing agents that tend to promote healing and, possibly, lessen the pain.[41]

Melissa (Balm)

An herb that has shown some promise in the treatment of cold sores is melissa. Consisting of the dried leaves, with or without flowering tops, of *Melissa officinalis* L. (family Lamiaceae), this fragrant herb has been used medicinally for more than 20 centuries. For most of this time, it was employed for its sedative, spasmolytic, and antibacterial properties. These effects are attributed primarily to a volatile oil, which is contained in quality plant material in concentrations of at least 0.05 percent. Some of the chief constituents of the oil include citronellal, citral a, citral b, and many other mono- and sesquiterpenes.[53] The German Commission E has found melissa to be a safe and effective calmative and carminative.[54]

It was first demonstrated in 1978 that an aqueous extract of melissa, containing a variety of polyphenolic substances, including oxidation products of caffeic acid and its derivatives, demonstrated antiviral activity.[55] The caffeic acid oxidation product is said to inhibit not only herpes simplex type 1 virus, which causes cold sores, but the herpes simplex type 2 virus, which causes genital lesions.[56]

A pharmaceutical product for external use is currently marketed in Europe for the treatment of both types 1 and 2 of the herpes simplex virus. It contains a concentrated extract of melissa representing 0.7 g. of the leaves per gram of cream-based ointment. Application of the ointment 2 to 4 times daily is said to shorten the healing time of the lesions and to decrease their recurrence rate. The preparation is not available in the United States, but a similar effect can be achieved by preparing a strong tea (infusion) from 2 or 3 teaspoonfuls (2 or 3 g.) of the finely cut leaves and about 1/2 cup

(150 ml.) of water. A pledget of cotton saturated with this solution should be applied to the lesions several times daily.

Much further research is required before the reliability of this remedy for treating cold sores can be assessed. Its efficacy depends on several factors, including the ability of the contained polyphenols to come in contact with the virus. However, untoward side effects of melissa have not been reported when used for this purpose. Further, the treatment is probably as effective as any other self-selected remedy for cold sores.

Dental Plaque

Plaque first develops on the enamel of a tooth as a thin pellicle of glycoprotein-mucoprotein derived from saliva. The pellicle harbors acid-producing bacteria that also form long-chain carbohydrate polymers causing it to thicken into plaque; if it is not removed, calcium salts in the saliva precipitate and convert the plaque into calculus or tartar. Bacteria in the plaque produce acids and other irritants that not only cause tooth decay (caries) but also inflame the gums causing gingivitis. If untreated, the gingival tissue becomes tender and bleeds, ultimately pulling away from the teeth and leaving pockets that can become infected, a condition known as periodontitis. Periodontal disease is now responsible for 70 percent of the tooth loss in the United States.[41]

Significant Herbs

Several herbs are incorporated into antiplaque dentifrices and mouthwashes. They function primarily as antimicrobial agents inhibiting bacterial adherence to newly formed pellicle and preventing it from being converted into plaque.

Bloodroot (Sanguinaria)

One of the most popular of these herbs is bloodroot. The dried rhizome of *Sanguinaria canadensis* L. of the family Papaveraceae contains about 4 to 7 percent of a mixture of isoquinoline alkaloids, about one-fifth of which is sanguinarine. Bloodroot was once widely used as a stimulating expectorant in various cough preparations; it also enjoyed a considerable folkloric reputation as a treatment for cancer.[57]

Sanguinaria extract, representing a mixture of the total alkaloids, has been incorporated into toothpaste (0.075 percent) and a mouthwash (0.03 percent). A large number of clinical and toxicological studies attest to these products' apparent efficacy and safety in the prevention of plaque and subsequent periodontal disease.[58,59,60] These comments apply only to the commercial bloodroot products when used in accordance with the manufacturers' instructions. Use of self-prepared dosage forms of this herb is definitely not recommended.

Minor Herbs

Some potentially useful herbs for the prevention of plaque include the leaves of:

Neem–*Antelaea azadirachta* (L.) Adelbert (family Meliaceae);
Mango–*Mangifera indica* L. (family Anacardiaceae);
Basil–*Ocimum basilicum* L. (family Lamiaceae);
Tea–*Camellia sinensis* (L.) O. Kuntze (family Theaceae); and
Curry Leaves–*Murraya koenigii* (L.) Spreng. (family Rutaceae).
In India, these individual plant materials are simply rubbed against the teeth to inhibit plaque formation and to treat periodontal disease. Limited in-vitro studies confirm the antimicrobial effects of the herbs, and some clinical evidence supports the utility of their aqueous extracts as antiplaque agents in humans. Neem is an ingredient in commercial toothpastes currently marketed in India and Pakistan.[61] Because of the preliminary nature of the clinical studies on the antiplaque value of these five plants, they are not necessarily recommended but are mentioned here as a matter of record.

REFERENCE NOTES

1. Robinson, J.R.: "Chapter 30" in *Handbook of Nonprescription Drugs*, 9th ed., American Pharmaceutical Association, Washington, D.C., 1990, pp. 811-819.

2. Wren, R.C.: *Potter's New Cyclopaedia of Botanical Drugs and Preparations*, rev. ed., C.W. Daniel, Saffron Walden, England, 1988, p. 285.

3. Osol, A. and Farrar, G.E., Jr.: *The Dispensatory of the United States of America*, 24th ed., J.B. Lippincott, Philadelphia, 1947, pp. 1563-1564.

4. Hänsel, R.: *Phytopharmaka*, 2nd ed., Springer-Verlag, Berlin, 1991, pp. 206-208.

5. Wichtl, M., ed.: *Teedrogen*, Wissenschaftliche Verlagsgesellschaft, Stuttgart, 1984, pp. 351-352.

6. Fowler, J.F., Jr.: "Contact Dermatitis" in *Conn's Current Therapy*, H.F. Conn and R.E. Rakel, eds., W.B. Saunders, Philadelphia, 1984, pp. 787-789.

7. Tyler, V.E.: *Hoosier Home Remedies*, Purdue University Press, West Lafayette, Indiana, 1985, pp. 124-125.

8. Lipton, R.A.: *Annals of Allergy* 16:526-527 (1958).

9. Bond, C.A.: "Chapter 33" in *Handbook of Nonprescription Drugs*, 9th ed., American Pharmaceutical Association, Washington, D.C., 1990, pp. 889-900.

10. Snyder, I.S. and Finch, R.G.: "Chapter 59" in *Modern Pharmacology*, 3rd ed., C.R. Craig and R. E. Stitzel, eds., Little, Brown, Boston, 1990, pp. 768-775.

11. Odom, R.B. and Rees, R.B., Jr.: "Chapter 4" in *Current Medical Diagnosis & Treatment 1990*, S.A. Schroeder, M. A. Krupp, L.M. Tierney, Jr., and S.J. McPhee, eds., Appleton & Lange, Norwalk, Connecticut, 1990, pp. 87-93.

12. Leung, A.Y.: *Encyclopedia of Common Natural Ingredients Used in Food, Drugs, and Cosmetics*, John Wiley & Sons, New York, 1980, pp. 24-26.

13. Fox, T.R.: *Health Foods Business* 36:45-46 (1990).

14. Winters, W.D., Benavides, R., and Clouse, W.J.: *Economic Botany* 35:89-95 (1981).

15. Schmidt, J.M. and Greenspoon, J.S.: *Obstetrics and Gynecology* 78:115-117 (1991).

16. Klein, A.D. and Penneys, N.S.: *Journal of the American Academy of Dermatology* 18:714-720 (1988).

17. McCauley, R.L., Heggers, J.P., and Robson, M.C.: *Postgraduate Medicine* 88(8):67-68, 73-77 (1990).

18. Fulton, J.E., Jr.: *Journal of Dermatologic Surgery and Oncology* 16:460-467 (1990).

19. *Lawrence Review of Natural Products:* June, 1988.

20. Ibid.: February, 1991.

21. Haas, H.: *Arzneipflanzenkunde*, B.I. Wissenschaftsverlag, Mannheim, 1991, p. 162.

22. Herrmann, H.-D., Willuhn, G, and Hausen, B.M.: *Planta Medica* 34:299-304 (1978).

23. *Bundesanzeiger* (Cologne, Germany): December 5, 1984.

24. *Lawrence Review of Natural Products:* September, 1987.

25. Wichtl, M., ed.: *Teedrogen*, Wissenschaftliche Verlagsgesellschaft, Stuttgart, 1984, pp. 274-276.

26. *Bundesanzeiger* (Cologne, Germany): March 13, 1986.

27. *Lawrence Review of Natural Products:* January, 1987.

28. Weiss, R.F.: *Herbal Medicine*, AB Arcanum, Gothenburg, Sweden, 1988, pp. 334-335.

29. Gracza, L., Koch, H., Löffler, E.: *Archiv der Pharmazie* 318:1090-1095 (1985).

30. Awang, D.V.C.: *HerbalGram* No. 25: 20-23 (1991).

31. Jaarsma, T.A., Lohmanns, E., Gadello, T.W.J., and Malingré, T.M.: *Plant Systematics and Evolution* **167**:113 127 (1989).

32. *Bundesanzeiger* (Cologne, Germany): June 17, 1992.

33. List, P.H. and Hörhammer, L., eds. *Hagers Handbuch der Pharmazeutischen Praxis*, 4th ed., vol. 5, Springer-Verlag, Berlin, 1976, p. 750.

34. Babny, P.: *Health Foods Business* **35**(7):65-66 (1989).

35. Penfold, A.R. and Morrison, F.R.: "'Tea Tree Oils'" in *The Essential Oils*, vol. 4., E. Guenther, ed., D. Van Nostrand, New York, 1950, pp. 529-532.

36. *Lawrence Review of Natural Products:* January, 1991.

37. Blackwell, A.L.: *Lancet* **337**:300 (1991).

38. Bassett, I.B., Pannowitz, D.L., and Barnetson, R. St. C.: *Medical Journal of Australia* **153**:455-458 (1990).

39. Garabedian, G.A.: *Science* **171**:847-848 (1971).

40. Hilton, E., Isenberg, H.D., Alperstein, P., France, K., and Borenstein, M.T.: *Annals of Internal Medicine* **116**:353-357 (1992).

41. Baker, K.A.: "Chapter 23" in *Handbook of Nonprescription Drugs,* 9th ed., American Pharmaceutical Association, Washington, D.C., 1990, pp. 653-675.

42. Berkow, R., ed.: *The Merck Manual of Diagnosis and Therapy*, 15th ed., Merck Sharp & Dohme Research Laboratories, Rahway, New Jersey, 1987, pp. 2322-2337.

43. Sollmann, T.: *A Manual of Pharmacology*, 7th ed., W. B. Saunders, Philadelphia, 1948, pp. 257-258.

44. Wren, R.C.: *Potter's New Cyclopaedia of Botanical Drugs and Preparations*, rev. ed., C. W. Daniel, Saffron Walden, England, 1988, p. 132.

45. Tyler, V.E., Brady, L.R., and Robbers, J.E.: *Pharmacognosy*, 9th ed., Lea & Febiger, Philadelphia, 1988, p. 151.

46. Wichtl, M., ed.: *Teedrogen*, Wissenschaftliche Verlagsgesellschaft, Berlin, 1991, pp. 238-239.

47. *Bundesanzeiger* (Cologne, Germany): August 14, 1987.

48. Weiner, M.: *Health Foods Business* **37**(8):16-17 (1991).

49. Keller, M.S.: *Mysterious Herbs & Roots*, Peace Press, Culver City, California, 1978, pp. 300-314.

50. Wichtl, M., ed.: *Teedrogen*, Wissenschaftliche Verlagsgesellschaft, Berlin, 1991, pp. 283-285.

51. Hänsel, R.: *Phytopharmaka*, 2nd ed., Springer-Verlag, Berlin, 1991, pp. 95-96.

52. *Bundesanzeiger* (Cologne, Germany): May 15, 1985.

53. Koch-Heitzmann, I. and Shultze, W.: *Deutsche Apotheker Zeitung* **124**:2137-2145 (1984).

54. *Bundesanzeiger* (Cologne, Germany): March 6, 1990.

55. Koch-Heitzmann, I. and Schultze, W.: *Zeitschrift für Phytotherapie* **9**:77-85 (1988).

56. Haas, H.: *Arzneipflanzenkunde*, B.I. Wissenschaftsverlag, Mannheim, 1991, pp. 148-149.

57. *Lawrence Review of Natural Products:* November, 1986.

58. Godowski, K.C.: *Journal of Clinical Dentistry* **1**(4):96-101 (1989).

59. Frankos, V.H. et al. (6 other authors): *Journal of the Canadian Dental Association* **56** (7 supplement):41-47 (1990).

60. Harper, D.S., Mueller, L.J., Fine, J.B., Gordon, J., and Laster, L.L.: *Journal of Periodontology* **61**:352-358 (1990).

61. Patel, V.K. and Venkatakrishna-Bhatt, H.: *International Journal of Clinical Pharmacology, Therapy and Toxicology* **26**:176-184 (1988).

Chapter 12

Performance and Immune Deficiencies

PERFORMANCE AND ENDURANCE ENHANCERS

Stress results when a person is overwhelmed by events and is unable to adapt to them. The condition may be induced by such factors as disease; inappropriate environmental factors; pressures associated with the workplace; inadequate rest; or other physical, chemical, or emotional factors that cause bodily or mental tension. Response to the condition differs for each individual, varying according to the subject's makeup and personality. It may involve anxiety, depression, fear, guilt, or many other subjective responses, as well as certain physical illnesses. Treatment may be behavioral, psychologic, social, or pharmaceutical.[1]

The herbal treatments used to increase resistance to stress are basically two: the ginsengs and eleuthero. Eleuthero is a relative newcomer to herbal medicine, having been introduced in the Soviet Union in the 1960s. Asian ginseng, on the other hand, has been used continuously in China as a tonic and aphrodisiac for centuries. The use of the word "tonic" in connection with both these herbs has generally been displaced in the herbal literature by the Russian-coined term "adaptogen." This has been defined as an agent that increases resistance to physical, chemical, and biological stress and builds up general vitality, including the physical and mental capacity for work. The Russian term has not been widely adopted in the standard English medical and pharmaceutical literature. It is extensively used in the herbal literature.

The Ginsengs

These consist of the dried root of several species of the genus *Panax* of the family Araliaceae. Asian or Oriental ginseng, extensively cultivated in China, Korea, Russia, and Japan, is *P. ginseng* C.A. Meyer, the most commonly used species. American ginseng is *P. quinquefolius* L. Another type, less frequently encountered, is san qui ginseng from *P. pseudo-ginseng* Wallich. There are qualitative and quantitative differences in the constituents of all three species, but in general, their effects are similar. Since American ginseng is little used here, being mostly exported to Asia, this discussion will center on Asian ginseng. It is the type that has been the most completely investigated.[2,3]

The principles believed to be responsible for ginseng's physiological activities are triterpenoid saponin glycosides, generally referred to as ginsenosides but also known as panaxosides. Asian ginseng contains at least 13 ginsenosides, each of which is designated by a capital R followed by a subscript letter or letter and numeral. Its exact composition varies according to the age of the root, the location where grown, the season when harvested, and the method of curing or drying. Because some of the pure ginsenosides produce effects directly opposite to those induced by others, and because all are present in the root in relatively small amounts, only the whole root, or a concentrated extract of it, is used in herbal preparations. In traditional Chinese thought, the whole root is more beneficial than any of its parts.[4]

Hundreds of experiments carried out in small animals have shown that ginseng extracts can prolong swimming time, prevent stress-induced ulcers, stimulate hepatic ribosome production, increase activity of the immune system, stimulate protein biosynthesis, prevent platelet aggregation, and induce many other effects, all of which might contribute to its general tonic or adaptogenic effects.[5,6] However, it appears fruitless at this time to carry out an extensive review of all of ginseng's purported effects in animals.

The problem with ginseng is that we are almost totally ignorant of its effects on human beings, at least insofar as results obtained from appropriate clinical studies are concerned. In 1985, Barna asserted that only one well-controlled experiment with ginseng in humans had ever been carried out, and its results were equivocal.[7] While believing that a number of well-controlled ginseng studies in humans have been conducted, Staba conceded that they have not yielded definitive results. He has also stated his opinion that evaluation of existing animal studies will not establish ginseng as a useful therapeutic agent. His conclusion is that long-term, controlled human experiments are needed to identify beneficial or harmful physiological effects.[8] Lewis has likewise concluded that ginseng has no proven efficacy for humans.[9]

Side effects of ginseng consumption attained some notoriety when they were addressed in a 1979 article by Siegel.[10] Because the paper appeared as a "Clinical Note" in the prestigious *Journal of the American Medical Association*, the results of the study were widely disseminated and have been extensively quoted in the herbal literature. He claimed that ingestion of ginseng could result in hypertension, nervousness, irritability, and similar side effects, which were grouped under a generic title, the ginseng abuse syndrome (GAS). Castleman, in a detailed analysis of Siegel's work, has pointed out that there was no control or analysis to determine what types of ginseng were being ingested, and further, some of the subjects were taking excessive amounts, as much as 15 grams per day.[11] Authorities now tend to discount the existence of a GAS, but Siegel's study continues to be quoted in the literature. On the basis of its long-term usage and the relative infrequency of reports of significant side effects, it is safe to conclude that ginseng is not usually associated with serious adverse reactions.[5]

Ginseng is certainly the most costly root; choice specimens with humanoid shapes retail for thousands of dollars. Incidentally, it is this similarity to the human figure that, based on the Doctrine of Signatures, provides the herb with its ancient reputation as an aphrodisiac. Commercially, ginseng is available in a variety of forms, including teas, capsules, extracts, tablets, roots, chewing gum, cigarettes, and candies. In some of these forms, it is extremely difficult to determine the quality and quantity of the root present. Experiments carried out in the late 1970s showed that 60 percent of 54 ginseng products tested were worthless and 25 percent contained no ginseng at all.[12,13] Whether the quality of the products on the American market has improved since that time is unknown. Since whole ginseng root is, with a little experience, easily recognized organoleptically, it is recommended that, to assure quality, the herb be purchased in that form. Alternatively, one must rely on the reputation of the producer or manufacturer.

In summary, ginseng has an ancient reputation as a tonic and aphrodisiac. Some supporting evidence for its effectiveness in such ways has been obtained from small animal studies, but significant data from controlled human trials are lacking. Those who choose to consume it for its purported effects do so in the form of a tea prepared from 1/2 teaspoonful (1.75 g.) of the drug taken 1 or possibly 2 times daily. Alternatively, capsules containing 250 mg. of the root are used. Ginseng preparations standardized on the basis of their ginsenoside content are available. Dosage is according to the manufacturers' instructions.

Eleuthero

The root of *Eleutherococcus senticosus* (Rupr. & Maxim.) Maxim. of the family Araliaceae was introduced into modern herbal practice some 30 years ago by Soviet scientists who were seeking a cheap and abundant substitute for ginseng. Everything possible seems to have been done to make this common plant mimic the scarcer ginseng. When various compounds were isolated from it, they were designated eleutherosides, a name resembling ginsenosides, even though they were not triterpenoid saponins but were sterols, phenyl-propanoid derivatives, lignans, oleanolic acid glycosides, and the like. When eleuthero was first marketed in the United States in the late 1970s, the name Siberian ginseng was utilized, further compounding the confusion.[14] In fact, so many people today confuse eleuthero with ginseng (*Panax* species) that knowledgeable persons almost universally refuse to use the Siberian ginseng designation and refer to the herb by its abbreviated scientific name, eleuthero.

As noted, eleuthero contains a series of unrelated compounds designated eleutherosides to which the physiologic action–tonic/adaptogenic–has been ascribed. The ginsenosides typical of ginseng are not present. No unusual compounds or any characteristic only of eleuthero have been detected.

Eleuthero is often misidentified or adulterated. In 1990, a case in Canada was reported in which a product labeled Siberian ginseng, initially confused with ginseng by the attending physicians, was subsequently determined to be the bark of silk vine (*Periploca sepium* Bunge of the family Asclepiadaceae), an herb used in traditional Chinese medicine.[15] Another sample of so-called Siberian ginseng, which did consist of eleuthero, was adulterated by the addition of 0.5 percent caffeine, presumably to provide a stimulant effect to the user.[16]

Almost all of the studies dealing with the biologic effects of eleuthero have appeared in the Russian literature. According to the summary by Farnsworth and colleagues, studies conducted on a total of 2,100 human subjects with no pathology were designed to determine the ability of humans to withstand various adverse conditions and to improve work output and athletic performance. Male and female subjects from 19 to 72 years of age were given a 33 percent alcoholic extract of eleuthero 1 to 3 times daily for periods up to 60 days.[17] The results were generally positive, and no side effects were reported. Another group of studies involved 2,200 human patients suffering from various pathological conditions including diabetes, hypertension, cancer, heart disease, and the like. Measurable improvement was said to be effected in many cases. Eleuthero is widely recommended for, and utilized by, athletes in this country who are told that it "stabilizes blood sugar levels during exercise" and "supports the body in adapting to increased levels of mechanical and biochemical stress that is induced from training and competing."[18] Some advocates fail to distinguish between ginseng and so-called Siberian ginseng (eleuthero). From the scientific viewpoint, it is apparent that most of the Russian studies of the effects of eleuthero on human beings were not double-blinded and also lacked adequate controls. Haas has concluded that the only effect of eleuthero that is adequately documented is that of an immunomodulator.[19] Weiss is also skeptical of the herb's utility.[20] Although capsules of eleuthero are readily available on the market, on the basis of existing evidence, its consumption as a tonic/adaptogen cannot now be recommended.

Sarsaparilla

Consisting of the dried root of various species of the genus *Smilax* that grow in Mexico and Central America, the technical nomenclature of these vining plants is extremely confusing. It is expeditious, therefore, to refer to them by the botanical origins assigned when the drug was last listed in the official compendia in 1965; prior to that time sarsaparilla had been monographed in the *USP* and *NF* for 145 years. Mexican sarsaparilla is obtained from

Smilax aristolochiaefolia Miller; Honduras sarsaparilla from *S. regelii* Killip & Morton; Ecuadorian sarsaparilla from *S. febrifuga* Kunth; and Central American sarsaparilla from other undetermined *S.* species of the family Smilacaceae.[21]

Originally, the botanical enjoyed an undeserved reputation for the treatment of syphilis. Later it began to be used as a flavoring agent both for pharmaceuticals and soft drinks (root beer). In recent years, it has been extensively advertised in body-building publications as a natural source of testosterone and a legal replacement for illegal androgenic steroids.[22] Some suppliers claim that sarsaparilla actually contains testosterone; others imply that it increases testosterone levels in the body following consumption. Neither assertion is true.

Sarsaparilla does contain several steroids, including sarsapogenin and smilagenin, as well as their glycosides (saponins), which can serve as precursors for the in-vitro production of various steroidal drugs. However, these compounds themselves do not function as anabolic steroids, nor is there evidence that they, or any other sarsaparilla constituents, are converted directly to anabolic steroids in the human body. Testosterone itself does not occur in sarsaparilla or in any higher plant.

As if this were not deception enough, it was reported in 1988 that for the ten previous years some commercial herb products labeled sarsaparilla contained instead *Hemidesimus indicus* R. Br., a plant sometimes referred to as false sarsaparilla or Indian sarsaparilla after the country of origin.[23] Belonging to an entirely different plant family (Asclepiadaceae), this substitute contains neither the same saponins nor the other principal constituents found in authentic sarsaparilla. The latter must be obtained from *Smilax* species originating in tropical America.

At present, the only legitimate use of sarsaparilla is as a flavoring agent. It has no utility as a performance or endurance enhancer. Because its utility is so often misrepresented, and another drug is often substituted for it, the facts concerning sarsaparilla are presented here as a matter of record.

Sassafras

Another herb that cannot be recommended but which is still widely used by lay persons as a tonic or performance enhancer and must, therefore, be mentioned is sassafras. As is the case with sarsaparilla, this native American herb, the root bark of *Sassafras officinalis* Nees & Eberm. (family Lauraceae), was originally recommended as a cure for syphilis. Although sassafras proved ineffective in this regard, it retained its ancient reputation, which became euphemistically expressed as a "blood purifier." In modern parlance, the herb is said to function as a tonic or performance enhancer; in fact, sassafras has been known to be without significant therapeutic utility for more than two centuries.[24]

Sassafras root bark contains 5 to 9 percent of a highly aromatic oil of which about 80 percent is safrole, a phenolic ether. In 1960, safrole was shown to be carcinogenic in rats and mice, and both sassafras volatile oil and safrole were prohibited by the FDA from use as food additives or flavors.[25] In 1976, bark sold for making sassafras tea was also banned. Nevertheless, the bark is still an article of commerce and is commonly, but unwisely, used as a pleasant-flavored spring tonic. For this reason, the herb is mentioned here, in spite of the fact that it is both unsafe and ineffective.

Ashwagandha

The dried root of *Withania somnifera* Dunal (family Solanaceae) is used extensively in Ayurvedic medicine as a tonic. Ayurveda has enjoyed considerable popularity in the United States during recent years, and several herbs used in its traditional healing practices are currently available in tablet form. Ashwagandha is one of these. Wagner and colleagues have reviewed the evidence supporting the herb's adaptogenic activity.[26] While preliminary tests in small animals indicate that several steroidal derivatives known as sitoindosides contained in the herb may produce some positive effects, substantial clinical evidence obtained from human studies is lacking. Until this is forthcoming, ashwagandha cannot be considered a useful adaptogen/tonic.

CANCER

Cancer is the second leading cause of death in the United States, producing some 400,000 deaths annually, particularly among older people where it predominates. The cancer (malignant neoplastic) cells are larger and divide more rapidly than normal cells; they serve no useful function. In addition, they metastasize, spreading by various means throughout the body from the primary site. Malignant tumors derived from epithelial tissues are known as carcinomas; those originating from connective, muscle, and bone tissues are called sarcomas.

The origin of cancer (carcinogenesis) has been intensively studied, but definitive results have not been obtained. It apparently results from complicated interactions of viruses, carcinogenic substances or conditions, immunologic factors, and diet. Some of the known carcinogens include radiation (the most dangerous), asbestos, aromatic hydrocarbons and benzopyrene, various alkylating agents, and tobacco. A high-fat diet and excessive use of estrogens have also been implicated.[27]

Because of its life-threatening nature, cancer is not a disease that is amenable to self-treatment. However, some plant drugs are currently used professionally in its treatment with good results, and others are recommended by irresponsible herbalists. It appears worthwhile, therefore, to provide a brief listing and discussion of such products.

Significant Anticancer Herbs

Catharanthus

The dried whole plant of *Catharanthus roseus* G. Don (family Apocynaceae), formerly designated *Vinca rosea* L., contains more than 70 alkaloids, two of which, vinblastine and vincristine, are extensively used in the treatment of a wide variety of malignant neoplasms.[28] Both of these alkaloids are prescription drugs requiring administration by a qualified physician. Because catharanthus is not employed in herbal form or as a phytomedicine, it is simply mentioned here to complete the record of plants, the constituents of which are successfully used in the treatment of cancer.

Podophyllum

Consisting of the dried rhizome and roots of *Podophyllum peltatum* L. (family Berberidaceae), podophyllum, or mayapple, contains about 5 percent of an amorphous resin sometimes referred to as podophyllin. Formerly employed as a drastic purgative, podophyllum resin is now used in the form of an alcoholic solution as a topical treatment for certain papillomas (benign epithelial tumors). Etoposide, a semisynthetic derivative of one of the resin constituents, podophyllotoxin, has been developed. It is administered intravenously for the treatment of testicular and ovarian germ cell cancers, lymphomas, small-cell lung cancers, and acute myelogenous and lymphoblastic leukemia.[29]

Pacific Yew

The bark of the Pacific yew, *Taxus brevifolia* Nutt. (family Taxaceae), contains a small amount (0.01 percent) of taxol, a compound that has been found to be very useful when administered intravenously for the treatment of advanced ovarian cancer. It appears that the principal problem relating to the drug is the scarcity of plant material from which it can be obtained. Studies are currently being conducted to identify other yew species that contain taxol, and tissue culture specialists are attempting to produce it in artificial cultures. Chemists are also working to synthesize the complex molecule or analogues of it. At present, taxol shows considerable promise of becoming a useful chemotherapeutic agent in the treatment of ovarian cancer.[30]

Unproven Anticancer Herbs

Phytomedicinals that have no proven value in the treatment of cancer but are nevertheless recommended for its treatment in the uncritical herbal literature are apricot pits, pau d'arco, and mistletoe.

Apricot Pits

Much less popular than they were a decade ago, the kernels of *Prunus armeniaca* L. of the family Rosaceae and their contained laetrile (up to 8 percent) or, more accurately, amygdalin, continue to be used occasionally as a cancer cure. An extensive clinical study begun by the National Cancer Institute in 1980 concluded that laetrile and natural products containing it were "ineffective as a treatment for cancer."[31] Apricot pits and laetrile are mentioned here only to call the reader's attention to their lack of therapeutic value.

Pau d'Arco

The bark of various South and Central American *Tabebuia* species (family Bignoniaceae) is sold under the name of pau d'arco, lapacho, or taheebo and used as a tea to treat various cancers. Presumably, it is purported to be effective because of its content of lapachol derivatives, yet lapachol itself was found to be too toxic for human use in clinical trials.[32,33] The effectiveness of pau d'arco for the treatment of cancer or any other condition remains unproven and cannot be recommended.

Mistletoe

Because of their reputation as toxic plants, neither European mistletoe, *Viscum album* L., nor American mistletoe, *Phoradendron leucarpum* (Raf.) Rev. & M.C. Johnst., is customarily available from commercial herb supply houses in the United States. Both plants contain similar toxic polypeptides known respectively as viscotoxins and phoratoxins, as well as lectins (glycoproteins), and many other physiologically active constituents, such as tyramine, histamine, and flavonoids.[34]

European mistletoe has an ancient folkloric reputation as a treatment for hypertension, but in recent years much attention has been devoted to its potential antineoplastic effects when administered by injection. Between 1985 and 1990, some 60 articles on this subject were published in the medical literature.[35] Nevertheless, mistletoe's effectiveness as an anticancer treatment is moot in this country because suitable injectable preparations are unavailable here. In Europe, where they are available, their utility as nonspecific palliative therapy for malignant tumors remains unproven and is controversial. In addition, the German Commission E has also declared that the use of the herb to treat hypertension requires substantiation.[36] Because the risk-benefit ratio of European mistletoe as a therapeutic agent is unacceptable, the Bureau of Non-prescription Drugs, Health and Welfare Canada recommended that products containing it be removed from the market there in 1991.[37]

COMMUNICABLE DISEASES AND INFECTIONS

One way to combat communicable diseases and infections is to stimulate the body's own immune system to resist the unwanted microorganisms. In general, this is called immunomodulation. Specifically, when an augmented or enhanced immune response is required, it is known as biological response modification. The mechanism of immunomodulation is complex, and a rather daunting nomenclature has grown up around the various components and factors involved.

The main effector cells of the immune system are: (1) macrophages that engulf microorganisms, (2) T lymphocytes (T cells) that protect against intracellular diseases and cellular neoplasms, and (3) B lymphocytes that develop into plasma cells which secrete antibodies or immunoglobulins in response to certain antigens. The T lymphocytes are classified into three types, depending on their function: T helper cells secrete lymphokines that stimulate the activity of T killer cells; T suppressor cells control numerous immune reactions; and T killer cells produce tumor necrosis factor. In summary, T lymphocytes produce cellular immune responses, and plasma cells derived from B lymphocytes, by the production of antibodies, induce humoral immune responses. Macrophages secrete so-called monokines that influence all immune responses; lymphocytes communicate through the secretion of lymphokines.[38,39]

Biological response modifiers (BRMs) or immunostimulants may effect either the cellular or humoral immune system or both. They are nonspecific in character, producing general stimulation of the entire system. Because the response capacity of the immune system is limited, BRMs are more effective when used in conjunction with other chemotherapeutic agents and when the disease entity is quantitatively small.

Echinacea

Of all the nonspecific immunostimulants of plant origin, the most comprehensively studied is echinacea. This name originally referred to the dried rhizome and roots of *Echinacea angustifolia* DC., the narrow-leaved purple coneflower, but it was often confused with *E. pallida* (Nutt.) Nutt., the pale purple coneflower, and with *E. purpurea* (L.) Moench, the purple coneflower. All three of these native American plants are members of the Asteraceae, and in today's usage, are probably more or less interchangeable. *E. pallida* and *E. angustifolia* were the species long recognized in *The National Formulary*; presumably both were utilized in the popular echinacea preparations ("Specific Medicines") once marketed by the Lloyd Brothers of Cincinnati. At the present time, Foster advocates the use of *E. purpurea*, simply because it is the only species presently cultivated.[40] The numerous studies of the herb carried out in Germany have utilized primarily the overground parts, not the rhizome and roots, of *E. purpurea*.[41]

Other plants have often been fraudulently substituted for echinacea. At the turn of the century, *Eryngium praealtum* A. Gray, known as button snakeroot, was commonly employed. In recent decades, *Parthenium integrifolium* L., often called Missouri snakeroot, has been a particularly troublesome substitute. This tendency toward falsification is especially important to recognize because echinacea is generally marketed as a tincture (hydroalcoholic extract), and in this form, substitution is difficult to detect. In the absence of any standards of quality for phytomedicinals, echinacea preparations should be obtained only from suppliers with impeccable reputations for integrity.

Echinacea has no direct bactericidal or bacteriostatic properties. Its beneficial effects in the treatment of infections are brought about by its ability to act as an immunostimulant. It increases phagocytosis and promotes the activity of the lymphocytes, resulting in the increased release of tumor necrosis factor. Hyaluronidase activity is inhibited, and the activity of the adrenal cortex is stimulated. There are indications that it also induces the production of properdin and interferon. All of these actions tend to increase the body's resistance to bacterial activity.[42]

The exact identity of the principles in echinacea responsible for these effects is still undergoing intensive study. High molecular weight polysaccharides, including heteroxylan which activates the phagocytes, and arabinogalactan, which promotes the release of tumor necrosis factor, certainly play a significant role. Stimulation of phagocytosis is apparently also enhanced by components of the alkamide fraction (mainly isolutylamides) and by chicoric acid.[43]

An enormous literature on echinacea currently exists. Three major books with extensive references covering almost all aspects of the herb and its medicinal application have appeared since 1989,[44,45,46] With such a vast amount of data available, as well as a great deal of information and misinformation in the popular herbal literature, it is difficult to summarize briefly and accurately the medical applications of the herb. Since neither the injectable nor the ointment form, both of which are utilized in Europe, is generally available in the United States, these remarks will be limited to use of the hydroalcoholic extract. It is generally consumed orally but may also be applied locally.

Oral consumption seems to be utilized primarily, but not exclusively, for preventing and treating the common cold and its associated conditions, such as sore throat. Preparations of the fresh overground parts of *E. purpurea* have been approved by the German Commission E as a supportive measure in the treatment of recurring respiratory and urinary tract infections. The words "supportive measure" denote that it would ordinarily be administered together with other antibacterial agents, antibiotics, sulfas, and the like. The Commission also has approved its local application for the treatment of hard-to-heal superficial wounds.[47] Preparations of the underground parts of other *Echinacea* spp. apparently are similarly useful in all of these conditions. Echinacea's value in the treatment of other conditions, including yeast infections, side effects of radiation therapy, rheumatoid arthritis, cancer, etc., although often extolled in modern herbals intended for popular consumption, remains unproven.[48]

Dosage of echinacea is dependent on the potency of the particular sample or preparation utilized. The producer of a typical American hydroalcoholic preparation recommends 15 to 30 drops (0.75-1.5 ml.) 2 to 5 times daily. The German Commission E recommends 8 to 9 ml. daily of the juice of the overground portions of the plant, or equivalent amounts of preparations made from it. In the United States, the former official dose of the rhizome and roots was 1 g. per day. Capsules containing it in powdered form are available. A decoction prepared by simmering 2 teaspoonfuls (ca. 4 g.) of the coarsely powdered herb in a cup (240 ml.) of boiling water is sometimes used, but is not recommended because not all of the active constituents are water soluble.[49]

In a personal communication to C. Hobbs, R. Bauer has indicated that some persons in Germany believe echinacea works by stimulating lymphatic tissue in the mouth, thereby initiating an immune response.[44] Although evidence in support of this assertion is scanty, if true it would support the use of a hydroalcoholic solution as the preferred dosage form. It would also suggest that such preparations would be more effective if held in the mouth for a period of time prior to swallowing.

Echinacea should not be used by persons suffering from severe systemic illnesses such as tuberculosis, leukosis, collagen diseases, multiple sclerosis, and the like. Commission E recommends that neither internal nor external use should exceed a period of 8 successive weeks.[47] Infrequent allergies may occur, especially in patients allergic to members of the sunflower family (Asteraceae).

REFERENCE NOTES

1. Brophy, J.J.: "Chapter 19" in *Current Medical Diagnosis & Treatment 1990*, S.A Schroeder, M.A. Krupp, L.M. Tierney, Jr., and S.J. McPhee, eds., Appleton & Lange, Norwalk, Connecticut, 1990, pp. 710-714.

2. Foster, S.: *Asian Ginseng:* Panax ginseng, Botanical Series No. 303, American Botanical Council, Austin, Texas, 1991, 7 pp.

3. Foster, S.: *American Ginseng:* Panax quinquefolius, Botanical Series No. 308, American Botanical Council, Austin, Texas, 1991, 8 pp.

4. Chandler, R.F.: *Canadian Pharmaceutical Journal* **121**:36-38 (1988).

5. *Lawrence Review of Natural Products:* March, 1990.

6. Wren, R.C.: *Potter's New Cyclopaedia of Botanical Drugs and Preparations*, rev. ed., C.W. Daniel, Saffron Walden, England, 1988, pp. 129-130.

7. Barna, P.: *Lancet* **II**:548 (1985).

8. Staba, E.J.: *Lancet* **II**:1309-1310 (1985).

9. Lewis, W.H.: "Chapter 15" in *Plants in Indigenous Medicine & Diet: Biobehavioral Approaches*, N.L. Etkin, ed., Redgrave Publishing, Bedford Hills, New York, 1986, pp. 290-305.

10. Siegel, R.K.: *Journal of the American Medical Association* **241**:1614-1615 (1979).

11. Castleman M.: *The Herb Quarterly* No. 48:17-24 (1990).

12. Liberti, L.E. and Der Marderosian, A.: *Journal of Pharmaceutical Sciences* **67**:1487-1489 (1978).

13. Ziglar, W.: *Whole Foods* **2**(4):48-53 (1979).

14. Foster, S.: *Siberian Ginseng:* Eleutherococcus senticosus, Botanical Series No. 302, American Botanical Council, Austin, Texas, 1991, 7 pp.

15. Awang, D.V.C.: *Journal of the American Medical Association* **266**:363 (1991).

16. Awang, D.V.C.: Personal communication, May 21, 1991.

17. Farnsworth N.R., Kinghorn, A.D., Soejarto, D.D., and Waller, D.P.: "Chapter 5" in *Economic and Medicinal Plant Research*, vol. 1, H. Wagner, H. Hikino, and N.R. Farnsworth, eds., Academic Press, Orlando, Florida, 1985, pp. 155-215.

18. Reaves, W.: *Health Foods Business* **37**(3):56-60 (1991).

19. Haas, H.: *Arzneipflanzenkunde*, B.I. Wissenschaftsverlag, Mannheim, 1991, pp. 135-136.

20. Weiss, R.F.: *Herbal Medicine*, AB Arcanum, Gothenburg, Sweden, 1988, p. 177.

21. Tyler, V.E., Brady, L.R., and Robbers, J.E.: *Pharmacognosy*, 9th ed., Lea & Febiger, Philadelphia, 1988, p. 486.

22. Tyler, V.E.: *Nutrition Forum* **5**:23 (1988).

23. Blumenthal, M.: *Health Foods Business* **34**(4):58 (1988).

24. Tyler, V.E.: "Some Potentially Useful Drugs Identified in a Study of Indiana Folk Medicine," in *Folklore and Folk Medicines*, J. Scarborough, ed., American Institute of the History of Pharmacy, Madison, Wisconsin, 1987, pp. 98-109.

25. Crellin, J.K. and Philpott, J.: *Herbal Medicine Past and Present*, vol. 2, Duke University Press, Durham, North Carolina, 1990, p. 25.

26. Wagner, H., Nörr, H., and Winterhoff, H.: *Zeitschrift für Phytotherapie* **13**:42-54 (1992).

27. *Professional Guide to Diseases*, 3rd ed., Springhouse, Springhouse, Pennsylvania, 1989, pp. 38-44.

28. Tyler, V. E., Brady, L. R., and Robbers, J. E.: *Pharmacognosy*, 9th ed., Lea & Febiger, Philadelphia, 1988, pp. 225-228.

29. Sikic, B.I.: "Chapter 61" in *Modern Pharmacology*, 3rd ed., C.R. Craig and R.E. Stitzel, eds., Little, Brown, Boston, 1990, pp. 818-819.

30. *Lawrence Review of Natural Products:* August, 1991.

31. Moertel, C.G. et al. (9 other authors): *New England Journal of Medicine* **306**:201-236 (1982).

32. Girard, M. et al. (5 other authors): *Journal of Natural Products* **51**:1023-1024 (1988).

33. Block, J.B., Serpick, A.A., Miller, W., and Wiernik, P.H.: *Cancer Chemotherapy Reports* (Part 2) **4**(4):27-28 (1974).

34. Schilcher, H.: *Deutsche Apotheker Zeitung* **127**:1268-1271 (1987).

35. Bowman, I.A.: *Texas Heart Institute Journal* **17**:310-314 (1990).

36. *Bundesanzeiger* (Cologne, Germany): December 5, 1984.

37. Kasparek, M.C.: Personal communication, February 11, 1991.

38. Wierda, D. and Reasor, M.J.: "Chapter 62" in *Modern Pharmacology*, 3rd ed., C.R. Craig and R. E. Stitzel, eds., Little, Brown, Boston, 1990, pp. 821-826.

39. Haas, H.: *Arzneipflanzenkunde*, B.I. Wissenschaftsverlag, Mannheim, 1991, pp. 133-134.

40. Foster, S.: *Health Foods Business* **37**(1):26-27 (1991).

41. Foster, S.: *Echinacea:* The Purple Coneflowers, Botanical Series No. 301, American Botanical Council, Austin, Texas, 1991, 7 pp.

42. Haas, H.: *Arzneipflanzenkunde*, B. I. Wissenschaftsverlag, Mannheim, 1991, pp. 134-135.

43. Bauer, R., Remiger, P., Jurcic, K., and Wagner, H.: *Zeitschrift für Phytotherapie* **10**:43-48 (1989).

44. Hobbs, C.: *The Echinacea Handbook*, Eclectic Medical Publications, Portland, Oregon, 1989, 118 pp.

45. Bauer, R. and Wagner, H.: *Echinacea: Handbuch für Ärzte, Apotheker und andere Naturwissenschaftler*, Wissenschaftliche Verlagsgesellschaft, Stuttgart, 1990, 182 pp.

46. Foster, S.: *Echinacea: Nature's Immune Enhancer*, Healing Arts Press, Rochester, Vermont, 1991, 150 pp.

47. *Bundesanzeiger* (Cologne, Germany): March 2, 1989.

48. Castleman, M.: *The Healing Herbs*, Rodale Press, Emmaus, Pennsylvania, 1991, pp. 150-154.

49. Castleman, M.: *Medical Selfcare* No. **53**:53-54 (1989).

Index

Abortifacient, 76
Abrasions. *See* Wounds
Acetaminophen, 127
Acetylsalicylic acid, 25
Acne, 157,160
Acorus calamus, 60
Acupuncture, 10
Adaptogen, 17,171-175
  ashwagandha as, 177
  eleuthero as, 171,174-175
  ginseng as, 17,171-174
Adhesins, 80
Adonis, 102
Adonis vernalis, 102
Adrenal cortex, 182
Adulteration, 4,5,18
Aescin, in horse chestnut seed,
  112-113
Aesculus glabra, 112
Aesculus hippocastanum,
  112
African ginger, 40
AIDS, 124
Ajoenes, in garlic, 105
Albuminuria, 77
Alcoholic beverages, 29
Alexandria senna, 49
Alkaloids, 29,119,128,139,158,162,
  166
  belladonna, 65
  of cinchona, 29
  of ergot, 29,128
  harmala-type indole, 119
  isoquinoline, 162,166
  of opium, 29
  pyrrolizidine, 139,158
Allantoin, in comfrey, 158
Allergens, 87

Allergic reactions, 57,58,108,110,
  157,184
Allicin, in garlic, 105,107
  activities of, 105-107
Alliin, in garlic, 105,106
Alliinase, in garlic, 105,106
Allium sativum, 104
Allyl isothiocyanate. *See* Volatile
  mustard oil
Aloe (Aloes), 50,51,155-157
  confusion with gel, 50,155
  description, 50,155
  efficacy of, 156
  Swedish Bitters, 51
  use, 50,155-157
Aloë africana, 50
Aloë barbadensis, 50,155
Aloë ferox, 50
Aloe gel. *See* Aloe
Aloë spicata, 50
Aloe vera. *See* Aloe
Aloë vera, 50,155
Aloë vulgaris, 155
Aloin A and B, 50
Alternative medicine, 10
Althaea officinalis, 92
Amabilene, in borage seed oil, 139
Amanita mushroom poisoning, 63,64
Amarogentin, 44,45
  in centaury, 45
  in gentian, 44
Amenorrhea, 137
American Botanical Council, 24
American Dental Association, 130
American ginseng. *See* Ginseng
American horse chestnut. *See* Horse
  chestnut seed
American Indians, 130,162

Steroids, androgenic, 176
Stimulants, 17,46,140
   action of, 46
   ginseng as, 17
   muscle, raspberry leaves as, 140
Stomachic, ginseng as, 17
Stomatitis, 161
Streptococcal infections, 98
Streptococcus thermophilus, 160
Stress, 171-175
Strophanthus, 102
Strophanthus hispidus, 102
Strophanthus kombé, 102
Substance P, in capsaicin, 125
Sulfa drugs, 79, 183
   and bearberry, 79
   with echinacea, 183
Sulfanilamide, Elixir, 19
Sunburn, 154
Sunflower, 184
Surface-tension modifiers, 97 98
Swedish Bitters, 51
Sweet birch oil, 147
Swertia chirata, 45
Symphytum × *uplandicum*, 158
Symphytum asperum, 158
Symphytum officinale, 158
Syphilis, 176,177
Syzgium aromaticum, 129

Tabebuia species, 180
Tachycardia, 39,131,140
Tachyphylaxis, 128
Taheebo, 180
Tanacetum parthenium, 126
Tannin-containing herbs, for
   dermatitis, 151-153
Tannins, 51-52,74,79,125,151,152,
   153,163,164
   astringent action, 51-52
   in bearberry, 79
   efficacy for diarrhea, 51-52
   in English walnut leaves, 153
   in goldenrod, 74

   in oak bark, 152
   in rhatany, 163
   in sage, 164
   in willow bark, 125
   in witch hazel leaves, 151
Taraxacum officinale, 63
Taxaceae, 179
Taxol, 33, 179
Taxus brevifolia, 179
Tea, 2,3,11,87,128,167
   anise, 60
   blackberry, 52
   blueberry, 52
   boldo, 62
   calendula, 157
   caraway, 60
   catnip, 121
   chamomile, 58
   comfrey, 159
   coriander, 60
   eucalyptus, 97
   fennel, 60
   horehound, 96
   marshmallow root, 92
   milk thistle, 64
   Mormon, 88
   mullein flowers, 92
   nettle root & leaves, 84
   passion flower, 119
   peppermint, 57
   raspberry, 52,139
   St. John's wort, 122
   saw palmetto, 83
   senna, 50
   thyme, 96
   valerian, 119
   willow bark, 144-146
Tea tree oil, 160
Terpenoids, in chamomile, 58
Terpinene, in tea tree oil, 160
Testicular cancer . *See* Cancer
Testosterone, 81-83,84,176
Tetracycline, 2
Tetrahydroberberine, in goldenseal,
   162